W9-AAF-523

THE GOSPEL OF GOOD SUCCESS

A Road Map to
Spiritual, Emotional, and Financial Wholeness

KIRBYJON H. CALDWELL

with Mark Seal

SIMON & SCHUSTER

SIMON & SCHUSTER
Rockefeller Center
1230 Avenue of the Americas
New York, NY 10020

Copyright © 1999 by Kirbyjon H. Caldwell
All rights reserved,
including the right of reproduction
in whole or in part in any form.

SIMON & SCHUSTER and colophon are
registered trademarks of Simon & Schuster Inc.

Designed by Ruth Lee

Manufactured in the United States of America

3 5 7 9 10 8 6 4 2

Library of Congress Cataloging-in-Publication Data
Caldwell, Kirbyjon.
The gospel of good success : a road map to spiritual, emotional,
and financial wholeness / Kirbyjon H. Caldwell with Mark Seal.
p.   cm.
1. Success—Religious aspects—Christianity. 2. Christian life—
Methodist authors. I. Seal, Mark, date. II. Title.
BV4598.3.C34   1999
248.4—dc21   98-43542
CIP

ISBN 0-684-83668-8

To my exemplary wife, Suzette, who has been my "Babi" since May 26, 1991, and who provided sensational encouragement and advice during the production of this book.

To our son, Kirbyjon Turner, who has helped to perfect my personal wholeness as both a husband and a father since November 14, 1997.

To my mom and dad, who have loved me healthily and unconditionally since August 4, 1953.

To my sister Dorothea, my brother-in-law Anthony, and my nieces Benaye and Nicole, who surround me with steadfast support and affirmation.

To Debbye, my sister-in-law; my grandmothers, Mama Josie and Mama Gussie; my in-laws, Papa Turner and Irene; and all my aunts, uncles, and cousins.

To the memory of my mother-in-law, Gussie L. Turner, who prayed my mom "back to life" when she was clinically dead for ninety minutes, who coordinated the family reunion in Jonesboro, Arkansas, where The Power Center vision was born, and who accepted me as her son prior to her death.

To the memory of my counselor, Curtis Tutson; my choreographer, Leory Hall; and my coach, Sherman Stimley—all of whom passed away tragically during the production of this book.

To the memory of my grandfathers, Kirby Hines and John Caldwell, for whom I was named, and my grandmother, Dorethea Hines, who showed me the way.

Contents

Introduction

THE MIRACLE

Beloved, I pray that you may prosper in all things and be in health, just as your soul prospers.
—3 JOHN 2

This book of the law shall not depart from your mouth, but you shall meditate in it day and night, that you may observe to do according to all that is written in it. For then will you make your way prosperous, and then you will have good success.
—JOSHUA 1:8

IMAGINE YOURSELF IN A HOUSE OF WORSHIP, DOESN'T MATTER which denomination or whether it is affiliated with a denomination at all. Just imagine some holy place, bathed in sunlight on some flawless Sunday morning. Things begin slowly before gradually rising in a crescendo. You watch the choir setting up, the congregation filing in, the background noise of muffled conversation, shuffling prayer-book pages, and building anticipation. Then the pastor or any other variety of clergy walks onto the pulpit. Strictly for the purpose of this daydream, allow that person to be me, Kirbyjon H. Caldwell, pastor of Windsor Village United Methodist Church, in Houston, Texas, one of the fastest-growing Churches in America.

"Good morning," I begin. "Thanks for coming. We have come here to praise the Lord."

The words serve as a cue for a mighty choir behind me, a ninety-member vocal cyclone whose voices rise up in sweet tones of exultation, singing, *"We've come to praise You!"*

But I'm not here strictly for praise. I'm here to talk about some bone-deep, dead-serious truth. Not truth about the world of the hereafter, but an entrepreneurial gospel of how you can maximize your God-given potential in the here-and-now. I'm here to help you identify the Faith within you that, once nourished, can rocket your life to new levels of empowerment and *good* success.

You might do a double take when you first see me in the pulpit. Because I don't preach in some regal vestment, not even a suit or a tie. I'm wearing a casual shirt and slacks. Expensive clothes are not a prerequisite to celebrating the Holy Spirit's presence at the church that you have just entered. We're here for empowerment, not posing. Any social barriers that might prevent people from feeling comfortable are barred at our door. I hope you've dressed casually too. Because now I'm directing 100 percent of my energy upon *you*.

Yes, *you*. Maybe you want a little more out of life—or maybe you want a whole lot more. Maybe you're seeking a more joyful life, a more satisfying career, deeper relationships, more money in the bank, better parenting skills, a more solid spiritual connection, a more healthy body, and a more muscular mental resolve. Or maybe your needs go deeper. Maybe you're sick, lonely, battling addictions, frustrated, suffering disease, battling low self-esteem, adrift in life. But if you're thinking God simply offers some pie-in-the-sky Sunday religious promise without regard to the realities of a Stormy Monday, you are about to discover a whole new world!

After all, you are a V.I.P. Like any normal person, you're seeking answers to three of life's most basic questions:

Value: What am I doing with my life that makes a difference?

Identity: Who am I?

Purpose: Why am I here?

Suddenly, the sunlight explodes through those stained-glass windows, the choir lifts its collective voice in awesome exultation, and you've found yourself in the midst of a miracle.

"We've come to praise Him!" sings the choir, clapping hands and swaying back and forth, a force of ninety people all pointing their fingers directly at you.

Then a light shines down from heaven and you hear some startlingly good news: *God wants you to be successful!* God has literally laid all the bountiful gifts of the universe at your feet . . . and I'm not just talking about the traditional concept of spiritual blessings but redemption in every aspect of your existence: your emotions, entrepreneurship, career, finances, relationships, health, parenting skills, academic career, and more. You have been given the promise of a successful and absolutely abundant life, but you must stand up, claim it, and develop a strategy to attain it.

You're on your feet now, arms in the air, running down the aisle like somebody who's won the lottery or picked the right door on a TV game show. The people who matter most in your life— your husband or wife, mother and father, children, friends, and associates—are gathered around you, hugging you, congratulating you, wishing you well.

You have become whole in every aspect of your existence.

You have entered the place of Holistic Salvation, with special emphasis on that first syllable. *Whole.* In this place, there is no such thing as a halfway God—or a partial person. Here, God doesn't restrict his grace to your soul, but watches over every aspect of your well being. God doesn't bless you on Sunday, then turn a blind eye the moment you step into the streets. God's Salvation is available every day of the week.

Whole. Keep this word in mind throughout the reading of this book. It's the one-word essence of Holistic Salvation. Once you become whole within yourself and within God's preferred vision for your life, you have begun to position yourself in the aspired place of Holistic Salvation. All of the pieces of your life—your financial, emotional, relational, professional, physical, and spiritual pieces—will be in sync, not as pieces of some convoluted puzzle but as pieces fitting harmoniously together as a whole. You will be complete—ready, willing, and able to realize God's optimal plan for your future.

You might think the scenario presented above is a fantasy, but I've seen it happen over and over again at Windsor Village, where our worship celebrations are just as likely to end with a prayer for blessed social relationships or economic opportunities as with spiritual redemption. There is, however, one caveat: God is not a game-show host. God doesn't always offer instant gratification. God sets up a road to success, to Holistic Salvation, a road that can have as many ups and downs as a roller coaster, and only those willing to make the sacrifices of the journey enter the place where all your dreams line up with God's purpose for your life, whether it's an emotional state, a financial condition, or a spiritual transformation.

Now, I know what you're thinking: "Where's the road map, what's the fee, and where are we going?" Well, the road map is in this book, the fee is whatever price you put on persistence, and the destination is, as I mentioned before, a place called Holistic Salvation.

Let me take you there.

THE POWER CENTER

I have discovered in life that there are ways of getting almost anywhere you want to go, if you really want to go.
— LANGSTON HUGHES

If you want to see Holistic Salvation in action, come to Windsor Village, a Church whose membership has grown from 25 to more than 11,500 in the past sixteen years. At Windsor Village, we don't just preach about Holistic Salvation; we practice it daily. We're a lean, mean Kingdom-building machine, with over 120 "ministries," serving the community seven days a week. There are ministries for everything from job placement and financial planning to weight loss and alcohol rehabilitation, ministries for everything that will help somebody step out of the herd and become a leader of his or her own life.

The story of Windsor Village is prayer coupled with action, and proof of the incredible power of this combination stands one mile from our church: The Power Center, the name of our 24-acre, 10,400-square-foot multi-use business complex designed to address the multifaceted needs of our community. The Power Center is our Church's physical manifestation of Holistic Salvation: We actually "salvaged" an abandoned Kmart building and auto-supply store and turned it into a reservoir of empowerment, serving the community's needs culturally, economically, educationally, emotionally, medically, socially, and spiritually. The Power Center houses a private school, the Imani School, a University of Texas Science Center–Memorial Hermann Hospital health clinic, a Chase Bank of Texas branch office, a Houston Community College business technology center, a Woman-Infant-Children's (W.I.C.) center, which aids approximately 6,000 women and children each month, and a full complement of executive suites, individual businesses, the fourth-largest conference center/meeting facility in the city, and much, much more. *The Wall Street Journal, Newsweek,* the BBC, NBC-TV, and other media have hailed The Power Center as an entrepreneurial incarnation of the twenty-first-century Church. We got the idea from Wal-mart, a mega-market with everything under one roof.

Over the next few years, The Power Center will pump about $30 million into the local economy. It has already added 275 new jobs to the community. Most important, it meets the diverse needs of our community inside one building, bringing together the diverse pieces of life that we once had to go to dozens of places to find—which, in an important sense, is the essence of Holistic Salvation.

My mission in this book is to show you how to use the principles of Holistic Salvation to create an internal center of power in your own life. Just as God doesn't limit grace to matters of the soul, the power of Holistic Salvation is not restricted to the walls of worship. Holistic Salvation involves knowing that God wants you to be successful in all areas of your life and, armed with that knowledge and inspiration, to build a life that is the epitome of good success, as defined in Joshua 8.

To begin, you need to know where you want to go in your life. Yes, I know you're probably thinking that's not so simple. Well, using the principles of Holistic Salvation will help you discover God's primary purpose for your life and how to achieve it.

You Must Be Present to Win

First step to achieving Holistic Salvation? Congratulate yourself for getting this far.

I'm not kidding. You have something to celebrate. You've beaten some incredible odds. The fact that you're reading these words tells me that you possess the most important aspect of your ability to employ the principles of Holistic Salvation to find your Calling and follow your Vision into an incredible new realm of living:

You're alive.

That's one whale of a feat! A rare accomplishment! I frequently ask myself, "Why are you still here, Kirbyjon Hines Caldwell?" Why, when so many of the folk you grew up with, went to school with, or began work with are dead or dying, why did you survive? Why is God preserving your life? Why didn't you succumb to the growing statistics of doom that level our nation's population? What made that equal-opportunity destroyer—the forces that can snuff out a princess's life as easily as a pimp's—pass over your house?

By the time I was twelve or thirteen years old, I had been a pall-bearer in more funerals than I had attended weddings. My high school classmates and Church members have been weeded out like soldiers in a war. Here's just a small sampling of victims from my high school class:

Fletcher Carter: the wrong end of a shotgun.

Caroline Wiseman: sickle-cell anemia.

Gerald Guinn: car crash.

Chucksy Ferguson: complications due to cardiovascular surgery.

Recently, another boyhood friend died even more tragically. He had been in a car accident about eight years ago. He survived the wreck, but not the aftermath. He became a paraplegic. He never quite got over that. One Tuesday, during rush hour, he rolled his wheelchair out in front of an eighteen-wheeler on the 610 Free-way in Houston.

I could go on and on. Car accidents, drownings, suicides, drug overdoses, alcoholism, workaholism, unprocessed anger, cancer, brain aneurysms, self-destructive behavior . . . Death has an arsenal of weapons waiting to destroy you. Consider your own list of lost souls for a moment. Then ask yourself, *Why am I spared?* As painful as death is, it does offer at least one potential prism of enlighten-ment: Death reminds us of the wonder of life. Life is truly God's most precious gift. As the Nobel Prize–winning author Toni Mor-rison writes, "Your crown has already been bought and paid for. So put it on and wear it!"

Why have you been "spared?" It's up to you to determine the reason and live out God's primary purpose and promise for your life. God's promises of success are incomplete, however, without your faithful response. God may promise, but you must push. God may declare, but you must decide to pursue that Divine declaration. God may will it, but you must walk it out. In other words, God's supernatural power is maximized when it is coupled with your faithful application of your God-given ability. Remember this equation: God's supernatural ability plus your faithfulness to act equals success. Or as my Grandmother used to say, "God helps those who help themselves."

You don't have to always ask God for some supernatural move as some sort of proof that God loves you. That's like awaiting permission from General Motors every time you want to drive your car. Add one critical ingredient . . . *action!* Never allow the enemy of negativity to paralyze you. It's easy to focus on what you don't have. Step out on what you have.

I'm going to give you a step-by-step road map to the summit of Holistic Salvation. But for now, there are four preliminary steps to begin as preparation for the journey ahead. Before you can find your Calling, then follow your Vision, use these four steps as sort of a preamble, a house cleaning, a way of preparing yourself for the inner and outer growth that is yet to come.

1. Realize that God wants you to be successful, but it's your responsibility to learn and follow God's vision for your optimal future.

For a long time there was a gulf, a divide that eventually grew into a canyon, in my thinking between who I knew God to be and what God wanted me to have. I went to primary school and attended Church in the socially torn neighborhood where I grew up, in

Houston. On Lyons Avenue, the crooks seemed to have a disproportionate allocation of prosperity. The so-called "bad guys," the pimps, prostitutes, hustlers, and numbers runners were driving Cadillacs and wearing diamonds, while some of the "saved persons" appeared to be struggling. So there was a gap in my mind between "being spiritual" and "being prosperous." This was further underlined by some churchgoing folk who thought you had to be financially broke in order to be holy. "It's tougher for a rich man to ascend to the kingdom of heaven than for a camel to pass through the eye of a needle," they'd say, quoting—and misinterpreting— the well-known Biblical verse.

Then, when I was in the seminary, a powerful verse in Joshua 1:8 began to resonate in my soul: "The book of law shall not depart from your mouth, but you shall meditate in it day and night, that you may observe to do according to all that is written in it for then you will make your way prosperous. And then you will have good success."

I was floored. Lights literally went off in my head. *". . . you shall meditate in it day and night, that you may observe and do according to all that is written for then you will make your way prosperous. And then you will have good success."*

"Whoa!" I thought. "God wants me to be prosperous and have good success! God did not make provisions—whether it's stocks and bonds, nice cars and nice homes, or peace of mind, joy, and healthy self-esteem—for Satan's kids. God's provisions are for His children, if they're for anybody!"

Note that all-important qualifier: *Good* Success. Which is to imply that there is bad success. The pimps and the prostitutes that I used to know? They had bad success, if they had any success at all, because their work was illegal, immoral, and unscriptural, and they were taking advantage of somebody else. The robber barons of corporate America who embezzle money, fleece the gullible, and de fraud the innocent? They also have bad success. God wants us to have Good Success. That doesn't necessarily mean having a seven-figure income or five Mercedes and a Maserati. It means that you don't have need for that which God has promised. You don't have to go begging for bread, with your tail dragging on the ground and your hand stuck out, looking for love in all the wrong places. God is calling you to be the head, not the tail, crowned with glory and honor!

This realization can trigger a powerful mental realignment. If you don't believe that God wants you to be successful—if you never realize that God wants to you to have self-control and inner peace, have a decent paying job, go on vacation—you will intrinsically develop behavior patterns that will destroy your potential to accomplish those goals. In order to receive and maintain certain blessings in life, you've got to realize that God wants you to have them. It is important to give yourself permission to be blessed. Otherwise, handling success successfully will be a constant struggle. You can become a spiritual schizophrenic, feeling that you aren't deserving of material possessions, emotional empowerment, or spiritual stamina or, even worse, digging yourself into the rut of emotional and spiritual poverty and powerlessness. Furthermore, unless you believe God wants you to be comprehensively success-ful, you're less likely to ask for the revelation of and empowerment for Holistic Salvation. Asking someone for that which you are not certain she or he can provide is an absolute waste of time.

For example, did you know that the ownership of land is sanc-tioned by God? It's practically unscriptural not to own land. In the Old Testament, owning land was a sign of God's presence and blessing, a sign of safety. It could be actual land or emotional land. Sometimes your Promised Land is not something you can see, touch, and feel. Sometimes, it's a spiritual move, sometimes an ac-complishment, sometimes it's a healed marriage, sometimes it's an obedient child, a healthy self-image, or a healed body. The "cattle upon the thousand hills" of Psalm 50, verse 10, belong to the children of the Lord. In other words, because I'm a child of the Lord, I'm entitled to some cows. Not only is economic development okay with God, the Bible *encourages* us to go forth and prosper as well.

So the first baby step toward Holistic Salvation is to realize that God wants you to be successful—blessed with a bounty of Good Success!

2. If you want good success, you have to have some funerals.

You heard me right. *Funerals.*

You've got to bury everything that's holding you back. If God ordains the blessings of good success, and you're not reaping your fair share of blessings, then there are some things—or some bodies—standing in your way. Now, think about this for a minute. You know what those things are. You've got to bury that fear, bury that doubt, bury that funky, nasty attitude. Bury those old family habits that haunt your current relationships with your children, spouse, friends, and business associates. Bury that wicked tongue that likes to cut people up one side and down the other side when your energies should be spent on your own self-improvement. Bury that mind of double-mindedness. Bury that indecisiveness, that self-defeating belief that life is nothing but rough roads and miracles are reserved for the movies.

Some of us need to bury some relationships with "some-timy," parasitic, leeching so-called "friends" and, yes, even some family members. You can get a strong indication whether you are in a self-defeating relationship by asking a simple question: Is this person helping me propel myself toward God's preferred future for me or restraining me from moving toward that future? (This question is equally applicable toward business associates.) If you're in a relationship that is full of all sorts of headaches, hurt, setbacks, and danger, then you need to bury it. You cannot move consistently toward the summit of Holistic Salvation if you're carrying Satan's backpack.

Did I say *Satan?* Indeed I did! If you think that Satan is some cartoon character, just wait until Chapter 4. We'll devote a full chapter to Satan and his many deceitful guises. For now, know this: The devil is out there, waiting to trip you up. The devil wants you to become disgusted, disenchanted, discombobulated, and any other "dis" that he can think of. That's the devil's job: to "dis" you. To become qualified for success, you're going to have to do some housekeeping. You've got to open the doors on the devil's hiding places in your life and boot him out!

If you're always sucking up to what somebody else's expectations of you are, then where is your identity, where is your integrity? Where is your dignity, purpose, self-definition, and God-anointed power? Every now and then, it's better to stand alone than to blindly blend into the pack. In other words, it's better to be a lion, roaring alone, than a donkey, braying with the dirty pack.

Some folks' self-esteem is so low, they think so lowly of themselves, they do not *want* success—either for themselves or for you. Those are the folks whom you can ill afford inside your concentric circles of friends or associates. They will not only leech off of you if you're not careful, you'll eventually adopt their mentality. Then, your desire for excellence and your pursuit of goodness will begin to dull and you'll be ready to settle for mediocrity. And once you've settled in there, getting back on the path toward Salvation is tougher than ever. So get rid of those nay-sayers—*now!*

And funerals aren't just for people. Negative ideas and emotions from your past can hold you just as effectively without the benefit of arms. Somebody reading this book is still being held hostage by something that happened forty years ago. You cannot move forward if you're always looking backward. Learn from your past but don't allow your past to incarcerate you. Build upon your past; don't be buried by your past. You have to turn your back to the past and press on toward your high calling! Apostle Paul said, "Forgetting those things that lie behind, I stretch toward those things which are ahead."

This is not a rerun or a repeat! It's time for us to move on.

Consider these wonderful words: stretch, reach, press, strive . . . they're active verbs, lion words. Words of action and power. Now consider words like guilt and remorse and regret. These are donkey words, passive, mulish language that takes you nowhere—at least not to those places where a lion wants to go. Words that keep you sinking into the quicksand of yesterday. What's then is then. This is now. Your dark yesterdays can be transformed into bright tomorrows.

As it is written in the Bible, "He or she who puts their hand to the plow and looks back is not fit for the kingdom."

Say it loud: "Been there, done that. Thank you! I'm movin' on!"

3. Become qualified for success.

After you bury your excess baggage and begin to move forward, you have to ask yourself another question. Are you qualified for success? If God were to give you your Calling and you could discern God's primary vision for your future right now, would you be ready to receive it? Are you ready to handle success successfully? You may not know where you're headed, but this much you can know: Where you are right now is not where you're going to end up. Your life is dynamic, not static. I once heard a very accomplished seventy-six-year-old man say with utmost confidence, "My best days are ahead of me." Yes, he meant it and, because of his conviction, he convinced me!

You have to prepare yourself for success, so when that Calling comes—and, believe me, it will come—you'll be ready to make your move. "Impossibilities are merely things not yet learned," the writer Charles W. Chestnutt once said. His meaning? The only impossible things are those we haven't mastered—yet. And becoming a master requires some dues-paying time as a disciple.

These days, there's a big belief in instant gratification. We want it and we want it right now. Some of us believe that because we can microwave pizza, TV dinners, and turnip greens, we can microwave success the same way. But good success usually takes time. You want to tell other folks what to do at work, but you don't show up on time. You want to be a manager, but you cannot manage yourself. Somebody reading this book thinks they should be promoted on their job because they've "been there" a long time. Well, just because you've been there doesn't mean you're ready to move ahead, unless, of course, you're qualified. A person with fifteen years of experience may have had the same experience annually for fifteen years. Seniority does not automatically mean qualification.

If you expect to move up the food chain of life, you can't just wish for it. You have to be prepared. For some, that means education. For others, it means counseling. For others, it means learning how to influence people. For still others, it means alcohol or drug rehabilitation. "If you do what you've always done, you're going to get what you've always gotten," goes the well-known axiom. To expand your world, you have to not only know about the world outside your existence, but be prepared to step into it when that time comes. As motivational leader Tony Robbins once wrote, "Knowledge is one of the ways to break the shackles of a limiting environment. No matter how grim your world is, if you can read about the accomplishments of others, you can create the beliefs that allow you to succeed."

As an example of how qualification manifests success, let's consider the story of "Baba and the Marching Band," a fable played out in Miami, Florida, in 1997.

The Miami Central Marching Rocket was qualified. Oh, yes, the "Rocket," the name of the 260-member marching band of the inner-city Miami Central Senior High School, had honed its music to near-perfection with grueling three-day-a-week practices. Thirty minutes of each session was set aside to exclusively train for a faraway dream the band held in its collective consciousness: to be chosen as one of twelve bands out of 260 entries from across America to march in the mother of all parades, the Macy's Thanksgiving Day Parade in New York City. When the judges made their decision, the Rocket rejoiced. *The band had won a slot in the parade!* But then the band members discovered it takes more than talent to march in the parade. It takes a staggering $185,000 in expenses. That was a seemingly impossible number for these mostly African-American kids in inner-city Miami, many from low-income, single-parent families. The school's resources were so meager, many band members wore pullovers and sweatpants because of a lack of uniforms and others were still waiting on trumpets, trombones, and percussion instruments.

With a year to raise the money, the band members began beating on doors, holding fundraisers, seeking community support, selling chocolates door-to-door, performing for pay at parties, and practicing, always practicing. But after six months of work, they had raised less than $25,000.

Then, one night, a forty-member unit of the band was hired to play two songs for $400 at a bar mitzvah in a Miami hotel. Part of the job was to march through the ballroom. As the band crossed the lobby in their green-and-white uniforms, they caught a wealthy businessman's eye. Not just any businessman, but Foutanga Dit Babani Sissoko, who goes by the nickname of Baba. Once an impoverished, unschooled West African house servant from the edge of the Sahara, Baba had amassed a fortune, first as a gold miner, then in oil, casinos, and diamonds. Now he's perhaps most famous for giving his money away: grants to schools and hospitals, $1,000 tips to hotel maids, cash to the poor and homeless, exhibiting such generosity that a rock star in his home country of Mali wrote a song in homage.

Watching the band cross the lobby, Baba sent one of his assistants over to ask the band members about their performance.

"We're performing to raise money for our trip to New York," the band's administrator replied, explaining the $185,000 plight of the Miami Central Marching Rocket.

The assistant huddled with the businessman. "I would like to help," Baba said. The kids watched in amazement as he pulled out a checkbook and wrote out a check. Then, the assistant asked the band members to huddle around the businessman.

"Would anyone like to guess how much the donation would be?" asked the assistant who served as Baba's interpreter.

"A hundred dollars!" exclaimed one band member.

"Three hundred!" exclaimed another.

"No," the interpreter said. "Mr. Babani Sissoko would like to make a donation of *$300,000* to your band."

$300,000! "The roof went off the hotel," the band administrator remembered. The kids were so ecstatic they were jumping up and down, screaming and crying and hugging Baba. The businessman's assistants and bodyguards had to literally form a circle around him to keep the kids from smothering him.

When the Miami Central Marching Rocket blasted off in two minutes of Thanksgiving Day airtime on NBC, playing "Rhythm Is Gonna Get You" and "God Bless America," the band's national debut had made an important statement. "Our story sends a message we can all learn from," says band director Shelby Chipman.

"You never know who's around you or who might be watching. So always be on the alert, always be at your best, and most of all, always be ready. It can happen."

The Miami Central Marching Rocket was prepared for success, even though they didn't know when, or if, they'd be able to exhibit that preparation. They didn't wait on their travel money before they began their journey toward their march down Fifth Avenue. The "Paralysis of Analysis" gets you nowhere. Action is majesty. The band acted on Faith and continued marching forward in their dream, trusting that somehow, some way, if they were ready, the money would come. Sure enough, when their blessing arrived, they could stand up and seize it.

Because they were *qualified*.

4. When God calls, answer . . . immediately!

How do you respond to God's blessings once they appear?

You move immediately.

Deliver me from pin cushion, powder puff people who sit around waiting and expecting deliverance like a letter in the mail. People who sit on their Humpty Dumpty behinds receive whatever trickles down. Like Humpty Dumpy, they eventually fall off their walls of complacency—and nobody can put them back together again. Life is not passing out blessings for those who sit and wait. You have to get out on that battlefield and claim your blessings. You've got to step up to the plate and take what is rightfully yours.

Some of us have allowed the devil to rob us of our blessings because we sat on our Holy Humpty Dumpties, waiting instead of going when God said *Go!* If God hasn't answered your prayers, maybe it's because the last time you asked He answered, and you haven't moved on the answer you were given way back in 1985!

When you are blessed enough to encounter a Vision, give it the respect it deserves. Move on it *immediately*! It's not just about doing it, it's about doing it *now!* Because to wait is just as faithless as saying, "No!" when God says, "Yes!" If you're hesitating, you need to know why. Because if the devil knows and you don't know, then the devil knows more about you than you know about yourself and will know precisely which traps to set to best drag you into the hell of disillusionment and despair. Discovering and dealing with your "dark side" issues is absolutely necessary for Holistic Salvation. The list of former and potential success stories who imploded because of a lack of self-knowledge and self-discipline is disgracefully long. We will deal with this in subsequent chapters. But for now, know this: *You cannot allow the devil to know more about you than you know about yourself.*

I've discovered that there are two kinds of faith. One is what I call a "buzzard" kind of faith. Buzzards out in East Texas are always circling the sky, eyes on the ground, never the horizon, looking to feed off the dead, whatever is left over after something else has come along and made the kill. The second kind of Faith, the Faith that we need to instill in ourselves, is an eagle's kind of Faith. An eagle always gets first shot. An eagle never hesitates. An eagle doesn't waste its time on leftovers or residue. An eagle swoops in with precision and power. We should aim for the eagle's worldview, refusing to settle for mediocrity, insisting on getting the fresh blessings on the front end, not the leftovers on the back end. An eagle's kind of Faith is a real threat to the devil. A buzzard's faith is circumstantial at best. The choice is yours.

To employ another analogy: Optimal living is like buying an ice cream cone. You buy an ice cream cone at 12 o'clock and eat it right away, then you get to eat ice cream. You buy it at 12 and wait until 1 o'clock to eat it, then you've got nothing but a mess. What used to be ice cream is now running down your hand and dripping onto the floor. That's the way a lot of us treat our God-given blessings. We were given the miracle of life, the equivalent of a heavenly ice

cream cone of absolute potential and promise. But instead of lick-
ing it, we just let it sit there, some of us thinking, "I'll save it for
later." But the longer it sits, the messier it gets, until when you finally decide you're ready to eat your ice cream, there's nothing left
to lick. Your window of opportunity has shifted.

N*ow it's your turn* to step up and into the arena of life and claim your
birthright. You were born for a reason. You have a duty to yourself to
discover that reason and follow it to its destination. In the next ten
chapters I am going to take you on a step-by-step journey to the
Promised Land of Holistic Salvation—that place where you realize
that you are made whole, having access to everything God meant for
you to have and the potential to be who God has called you to be.
    Here's a brief summary before we begin:

Chapter 1: Finding Your Calling

If you're seeking your Calling, the "why" of your birth, the first
place to begin is your past. Here, many a signpost pointed toward
your optimal future—if you had only taken the time to look, think,
and listen. In the Spiritual Gifts Workshop given to all new members of our congregation, we have been able to help many people
find their talents, confidences, and eventually, their true Calling in
life. I'll take you inside this workshop and show you how to use its
proven tools and techniques to determine your Calling. First step?
Ask yourself what God wants you to do between the cradle and the
grave. When you align what you truly enjoy doing with God's To-
Do list for your life, then the alignment of mind, body, and soul—
or Calling—will occur. I'll also show you, through the example of
my own past, how to sift through the sands of memory for the gold
dust of a new and absolutely enriching life.

Chapter Two: Staging a Comeback

The place where you begin the journey to Holistic Salvation isn't always pretty. But that's reason enough to get up and go! Just as every grand mansion begins on the riddled ground of a construction site, your new and improved life must begin on whatever ground, however shaky, you're now standing on. No matter where you are in your life, you can begin anew by staging a Comeback, following the proven steps of counted-out boxing champions, faded film stars, and down-and-out Churches to spark a powerful reawakening and a fresh start. I'm going to tell you the story of the comeback of Windsor Village and the amazing Comeback stories of some of the members of our congregation.

Chapter Three: The Faith Walk

Now, you're ready to embark upon a "Faith Walk"—in which Faith combines with action in an incredible explosion of power—toward your dreams. In this chapter, you will learn of the power of Faith, a fuel that renders even the most high-octane gasoline obsolete. When you align your desire with God's preferred state for your future and walk confidently toward your dreams, the seemingly impossible becomes possible in startling ways. The Faith Walk will be made much easier with the knowledge that for every step you take, God takes two. I'll show you how to employ the power of the great explorers to take the leap and march confidently toward the future.

Chapter Four: Whuppin' the Devil

Once you find your Calling in life and embark upon a Faith Walk, the devil is going to appear in one of infinite guises to try and trip you up each step of the way. I am going to show you how the devil morphs and mutates like some wily disease and how you can "whup" the devil by cladding yourself with the most powerful armor known to mankind. Once you defeat the devil, you've got to kill some Giants. What's a Giant? Well, if the devil is both the source of evil and the subversive thoughts that stop us—fear, shame, embarrassment, self-doubt—then Giants are all the actual things that we don't do because we think that we can't: seemingly unattainable goals, unfinished objectives, unfulfilled dreams. Revealing the seven attributes of Giant Killers, I'll show you how to become a modern-day David, killing Goliaths daily.

Chapter Five: Creating Wealth God's Way

More than half of the thirty-two parables told by Jesus in the Bible had to do with money. For an individual, or a Church, to deny the importance of economic development is like cutting off a plant from water. Today economic fulfillment isn't a luxury, it's a necessity. In this chapter, we're going to learn God's mathematics, a simple, yet practical formula for creating, and keeping, financial abundance in your life. I'll reveal the techniques we have used in our congregation to build everlasting wealth and explain how wealth follows those who discover their Calling and confidently follow their Vision.

Chapter Six: God-Blessed Relationships

"Love your neighbor as yourself" is one of the most powerful commands in the Bible. Now it can become the most empowering statement in your new life. Saying that you love somebody and knowing how to love them are two different things entirely. It all has to do with knowing how to meet each other's needs. To discover the sort of person you imagine as your optimal life mate, you've got to become what you want to receive. If you're married but unfulfilled, you must become everything you'd like your optimal spouse to be. If you're single but seeking, you must become what you'd like to attract. If you're single and wish to remain happily single forever, I'll show you how to continue to grow in your "oneness."

Epilogue: Becoming Whole

Welcome! You've entered the Promised Land of Holistic Salvation, the place where you're more than a sum of your pieces, but everything that God meant for you to be. This is not necessarily a place of arrival or rest or some sort of permanent pinnacle but the place where "new and improved" living can truly begin. Here's how to live and thrive there forever.

Now, put yourself back in that tabernacle of worship. Let the melodious voices of that choir cascade over you. And open your mind to the Gospel of Good Success. What you did yesterday is now ancient history. Action is power, and success is sanctioned by God. Let's take the first step into the world of Holistic Salvation.

1

Finding Your Calling

There are two great moments in a person's life: the first is when you were born; the second is when you discover why you were born.
—UNKNOWN

I BELIEVE WE ARE ALL BORN FOR A REASON AND IT IS OUR RE-sponsibility to discover that reason and redirect our lives toward God's optimal purpose for our lives.

It wasn't until I turned twenty-seven—after living for twenty-six fruitful, rewarding, experience-rich years—that I discovered the reason *why* I was born.

I hope to help you develop a road map toward your destiny in the next six chapters.

This is not an ordinary spiritual/self-help book. No book written by a former fast-track bond broker with a business MBA from the University of Pennsylvania's Wharton School, on the cusp of making more than $100,000 in 1978, who gave up his promising career to become a dead-broke, entry-level pastor, could be called ordinary. It's usually the other way around, isn't it? You know the stories: I-rose-from-living-in-my-storage-unit-to-running-a-multi-billion-dollar-corporation-in-nine-short-months! Not many authors would be excited about giving up a potential six-figure income and a job brimming with promise and possibility, a job that afforded me the new sports car, the power clothing, the unlimited potential . . . to become the pastor of a dying Church.

But something more than cash propelled me from one career path onto another, to discover a greater truth than I'd ever have known if I had kept my day job. It all started with a single recognition, a first step we all have to take if we are going to grow our lives from ordinary to extraordinary. It's something that we are given at birth but have to ferret out like a treasure hunter without the luxury of a map, something that can be the absolute starting gate of your new life, if you can only recognize it for the significance it possesses.

Now, bear with me a minute. Don't start moaning, "Oh, no, not another preacher talkin' about a Calling!" Really, when you think about it, every great achievement starts with a Calling, although I'm hesitant to even use the word. It's been abused and overused. Scoundrels go to prison and come out "Called." Public figures get in trouble with power, money, drugs, or sex, and emerge from jail or divorce court "Called." Criminals get "Called" right between the jury's decision and the judge's sentencing. Some folks have simply given the term "Calling" a bad name. Nonetheless, in order to begin the journey of Holistic Salvation, the word "Calling" is simply irreplaceable.

But I'm not talking strictly about a spiritual calling. I'm talking about a total reawakening, a Calling to realize your full potential in every aspect of your life. I like to compare a Calling to a lunar eclipse, only it's not the overlapping of the sun or the moon but the optimal alignment of your mind, body, and spirit with God's primary purpose for your life. When this happens, something will "click" within you, and you will know you've found your Calling. It's an instinctive, gut-level, spiritual experience. Prior to its occurrence, a Calling is a difficult concept to explain. It's something like Louis Armstrong's description of jazz: "Man, if you can explain it, you don't know what it is." You'll know it when you see, hear, and feel it. Until then, it's like a very dim light in a dense fog that you must follow until you find its source.

How to Find Your Calling

Frequently, the seeds of your Calling are in the simple reflexive things you do to compensate for some real or imagined shortcomings. The actor/comedian Robin Williams was a shy and studious only child, forced to spend his days alone in his parents' forty-room Michigan home. Usually only a maid would be in attendance. His parents were always away, his father on business, his mother doing charity work. His father was so distant, Robin called him "Sir" and "Lord Stokesbury, Viceroy of India." The boy so longed for a connection with his mother, he began using comedy to get her attention. "I'll make Mommy laugh, and that'll be okay, and that's where it started," he would later explain. He had found his Calling as a comedian. But if Robin Williams had spent his energies moaning and groaning, instead of releasing his frustrations on a stage, we would have been denied one of America's greatest comic geniuses. His sadness eventually led him to bring joy to millions of people—and to his success.

Think about it: Did you react to a problem—or declare a passion—in your youth that may have pointed the way toward your future? If so, write it down and begin thinking about it in detail.

Some of us are shown our Calling in our youth, but as adults we're required to take concentrated action on that Calling. This was the case of Sheree Perry, a member of our congregation. When she was a child, Sheree told anyone who would listen that she was going to become "a tomato lady." She's just always had a passion for food: cooking food, displaying food, discussing food. Knowing that cooking was her Calling, she grew up to be an incredible chef. But cooking alone couldn't lead her to the summit of Holistic Salvation, where her Calling would empower every aspect of her existence. She wasn't making any money from her cooking and, worse, she found herself in the middle of a divorce. Then, while driving on the Houston freeway one day, she says she had a revelation from God on how to turn her Calling into a career. She went back to school for courses in business management, and today she runs a lucrative catering operation. "The Bible says that God gives you authority over certain things," she says. "Well, he's given me the authority to cook. To taste my food is something that would linger forever on your mind. It's all the love that I put into it. It's just a powerful anointing."

Another child, another city. He was such a shy boy, he would routinely forsake the ordinary boyhood games to cling to his mother as she spent her days pursuing her passion—shopping in a discount dress shop. The boy's eyes would widen over the dresses that lured women like magnets. Back at home, the boy spent hours watching his *bubbe,* his grandmother, sew. The older woman had eked out a living taking in sewing after her husband abandoned her. The boy idolized his grandmother, and soon took up sewing himself, once even making an entire wardrobe for a doll that belonged to a friend of his older sister. "I never went through this thing most young people do," the boy would say later. "Going to school and not truly knowing what they want to do until later in life. I mean, I had a major head start—at age five, I had a pretty good idea of what I wanted to do."

The boy's Calling was clothing, and his name, Calvin Klein, has become a standard in the fashion industry for the past three decades. What initially made him different eventually made him great. Think about it: What makes you different? How could that difference be employed to propel you in a new purpose, a new meaning in your life?

Sometimes, your Calling can be revealed to you in a simple, single voice. You must hear the voice and heed its advice. That's what happened to Harry Wayne Huizenga, the garbage man. After returning to Florida following a stint in the U.S. Army, Huizenga was hired by one of his father's friends to drive a garbage truck in Pompano Beach. After a few years of driving that truck, a line that his father had repeatedly told him began resounding in Huizenga's head: "You can't make any real money working for someone else." Huizenga decided to take action on that advice. He started his own garbage collection company with a single truck and $500 in accounts, picking up trash from 2:00 A.M. until noon, then spending the rest of the day looking for new accounts. He became rich, first with his own growing garbage-collection company, and later, with the advent of the VCR, by building the massive Blockbuster video store chain. The garbage man had become a billionaire, the owner of three professional sports teams, and a model for entrepreneurs everywhere, and it all began when he heard and heeded words that he had been told for most of his life.

Finding your Calling opens the door upon the second step of the "why" of your birth. Because once you recognize your Calling and follow it to the place it ultimately leads, you will eventually gain sight of God's preferred future for you, a literal picture of what you're destined to do that's so bright and so unmistakable it's not merely a sighting: it's a Vision.

A Vision of who you can become and what you can do.

Perhaps the best example I can give you of the power of a Vision involves a man I first noticed sitting in the back row of Windsor Village one Sunday morning in the late eighties, a muscular African-American guy with a quiet yet powerful presence.

I had never even heard of the boxer Evander Holyfield, even

though he was a regular on Sunday mornings. Although he lives in Atlanta, his training camp is in Houston and he attends Windsor Village whenever he's in town. Later, he would even generously underwrite our new $1.2 million prayer center. But back then, I didn't even know his name until someone came up behind me on the pulpit and whispered, "Evander is here."

Warren Moon, then the Houston Oilers quarterback and also a Windsor Village regular, told me that Evander had boxed in the 1984 Olympics and had been disqualified on a technicality. "Now he's going to fight as a heavyweight," Warren said. "He has a chance to be a real good one."

As I got to know Evander, I discovered that one important aspect of his success as a champion was his ability to create a crystal-clear vision of where he was going. His vision came to him in a transcendent experience when he first met his father. The youngest of eight children, Evander never knew his dad as a kid. His parents never married. But they kept in touch, mostly because of the persistence of Evander's late mother, Annie. "I always promised myself that I would bring Evander back when he was grown," she would later say. "I didn't want him to think that he came from nowhere. I wanted him to know who [his daddy] was."

One day, Evander and his mother drove into a tiny Southern Alabama lumber town. There, Evander, a twenty-one-year-old cruiser-weight boxer wondering if he had the genetic material to grow into a heavyweight, stared at his father and saw a real-life Vision for his own future. The man was a broad-shouldered, 230-pound lumberjack big as any heavyweight. "It was a good feeling," Evander said later.

In that instance, when a twenty-one-year-old man met his estranged father, Evander Holyfield's Vision became clear: to some day fight for—and win—the title of Heavyweight Champion of the World. He could literally see his future standing before him. He knew from his father's size and heft that he had the ability to grow his body from cruiser-weight into heavyweight status. In that moment, Evander became a heavyweight in his mind. An ordinary circumstance became an extraordinary moment. A Vision was revealed; a future champion anointed.

Your equally transcendent moment awaits you, if you can only trust that someday, some way, your Calling and, later, your Vision will appear. When you discover not only who you are, but also *why* you have been born, then your hills are lower and your valleys are higher. Your journey through life will be smoother. That's not to say your rose garden is without thorns, but the trauma of travel is definitely minimized when you know where you're going—and why. Your life is no longer focused on defining yourself, but on traveling toward your destination. And on this journey, there will be some moments when the traveling is as enriching as reaching the destination.

Finding your Calling and a Vision for your future might take you a lifetime. But is it ever too late to discover what you have been born to do?

YOU'RE ON A MISSION FROM GOD

She figured she would remain a registered nurse forever. For almost ten years, she had risen in the ranks, from the lowest-level clerk to scrub tech to full-fledged RN, dutifully passing all the tests and doing all the work required, frequently coming home too exhausted to even remember why she initially entered the field. Sometimes, she would feel a pull from somewhere deep inside of her, a faint, faraway voice whispering three simple words: *"This isn't it!"* But she figured, "It's a job, it's a paycheck," and brushed off any thoughts of dissatisfaction with the dawn, as she trudged toward one more day in the life of a basically unfulfilling career.

If someone would have taken the time to ask her a simple question—"Is nursing your Calling?"—the nurse, the woman who had devoted her life to her career, would have had an immediate answer.

"No," she would have certainly replied. "But I'm too busy with the daily grind to pursue anything else."

Your Calling is nothing less than a mission from God. It's God's primary will for your life. It is the first step toward the Promised Land of Holistic Salvation. But while the process sounds simple, for many it remains extremely complex, a school of knowledge that education doesn't really address, a code that science has yet to crack. But it's something that is actually discussed explicitly in the Bible. *What were you born to do in life?* You were born to glorify God and follow His purpose. As we've discussed earlier, deep within all of us is a reason for our existence, a purpose, a Calling. Finding your Calling and following it is to not settle for anything but the best in yourself, and in the process, to glorify God and not to settle for anything less in your life. I believe that a true Calling involves three different aspects: first, the Calling glorifies God; second, it blesses, benefits, or helps somebody else; third, it brings you joy.

What were you born to do in life?

As a pastor, I have heard the question asked repeatedly, this central question of life. In our Church, we spend a lot of time identifying "Spiritual Gifts," God-given gifts, talents and confidences that the individual member can bring to serve God and our Church. But in discovering their Spiritual Gifts, scores of our members have invariably been led onto new and expansive career paths they could not imagine before. The philosopher Thomas Carlyle called finding our purpose "the first of all problems," and that's precisely what it is. "It is the first of all problems for a man [or woman] to find out what kind of work he [or she] is to do in this universe," Carlyle wrote. Work is the primary activity of living.

Like it or not, we spend more hours on our jobs than in any other activity. If the work that literally consumes your days is unsatisfying, unrewarding, and unfulfilling, then the other areas of your life will probably follow suit.

If you believe your career isn't connected to every area of your existence, just consider three of the infinite areas an unfulfilling life can destroy:

1. *Mental State?* "An unemployed existence is a negation worse than death itself, because to live means to have something definite to do . . . a mission to fulfill . . . and in the measure in which we avoid setting our life to something, we make it empty," the writer José Ortega y Gasset once wrote. "Human life, by its very nature, has to be dedicated to something,"
2. *Health?* "For many years, it has been known that job-related stress is a major contributing factor in a wide range of diseases," writes Laurence G. Boldt in his marvelous book *How to Find the Work You Love.* "It is perhaps not surprising, then, that according to the national Center of Disease Control and Prevention, more people die at nine o'clock on Monday morning than at any other time of the day or on any other day of the week. [Monday is also the most "popular" day of the week for suicide.] Recent studies have indicated that the greatest risk factor for fatal heart attacks is not smoking, hypertension, or high cholesterol (of which we've heard a great deal), but job dissatisfaction. Researchers at Columbia University have observed a link between coronary disease (the leading killer of American adults) and the individual's sense of control in his or her work life."
3. *Child Rearing?* The pioneering psychologist Carl Jung said, "Nothing has a stronger influence psychologically on . . . children than the unlived lives of their parents."

Not only was each of us born with natural talents and confidences, but through the gift of Salvation, we're also blessed with

something the Bible calls Spiritual Gifts. These are duties and attributes of the highest order which, properly employed, are intended to glorify God and bless one another. Realigning your life
toward your Spiritual Gifts—whether it's the gift of teaching, administration, wisdom, giving, hospitality, or, to be exact, twenty-
one other spiritual gifts—can rocket your life to an amazing new
level.

It's up to us to determine what those gifts and confidences are.
At Windsor Village, we offer all new members what we call a Spiritual Gifts Workshop, designed to help people find their specific
God-given gifts and, we hope, their Calling. Some of our members
pursue their Spiritual Gifts via involvement in a ministry. Others
experience such a revelation over discovering their gifts that the
revelation alters every aspect of their existence, especially their career path. We've discovered that the workshop basically confirms
what people felt they should be doing all along, even though they
had nothing on which to base those inclinations. They felt their
desires were dreams, when they could have been realities. When
your work becomes a labor of love, then it's not really work any-
more. But I've learned that vocational tests and evaluations cannot
compare to the power of a simple, single question, a question each
of us must ask and answer for ourselves:

Who are you and what were you born to become?

You have to know your mission before you can accomplish it.
You have to know your dream before you can achieve it. You have
to realize that somewhere, deep inside of you, no matter how
bright or how dim, is an eternal desire to do *something,* an absolutely
specific something. Through the haze of growing up and going
out, as we attempt to walk through the carnival fun-house mirrors
of parental desires, peer pressures, and career-consultant rap, amid
the chorus of voices all commanding us to *"conform!,"* in the blink
of the eye between childhood and adulthood, we forget, deny, or

never take the time to really realize what is it we were born to do. We look to parents, family, popular culture, want ads, or the marketplace of least resistance. We look everywhere, in short, except inside our souls, the place where the answers to our Calling reside. Some of us give up hope altogether. Some waste a lifetime drifting through dead-end jobs. Others settle for compromised positions, putting money ahead of dreams, and ending up eventually dissatisfied. Others accept whatever comes along in their lives without every truly seeing what could be. God is not glorified when people are systematically impoverished, sick, disenfranchised, oppressed, diseased, unemployed, begging for bread, ignorant, and/or broke. When your life is reduced to a fight for survival, you are denying your holy mission from God.

The proof of the power of finding your Calling is evident in any real success story. But one of my personal favorites comes from Norman Cousins' book *Anatomy of an Illness,* in which the author visits the ailing musical master Pablo Casals a few weeks before his ninetieth birthday. The maestro was in bad health: his wife had to wake him, help him dress, and lead him into the breakfast room. "Judging from his difficulty in walking and the way he held his arms, I guessed he was suffering from rheumatoid arthritis," Cousins writes. "His emphysema was evident in his labored breathing. . . . He was badly stooped. His head was pitched forward and he walked with a shuffle."

Before sitting down to breakfast, Casals performed a daily ritual: he sat down at the piano, arranging himself with "some difficulty on the piano bench, then with discernible effort raised his swollen and clenched fingers above the keyboard."

Then, Norman Cousins witnessed the medicinal miracle of a Calling.

"The fingers slowly unlocked and reached toward the keys like the buds of a plant toward the sunlight," Cousins writes. "His back straightened. He seemed to breathe more freely. Now his fingers settled on the keys. Then came the opening bars of Bach. . . . He hummed as he played, then said that Bach spoke to him here—and he placed his hand over his heart. Then he plunged into a Brahms concerto and his fingers, now agile and powerful, raced across the keyboard with dazzling speed. His entire body seemed fused with music; it was no longer stiff and shrunken but supple and graceful and completely free of its arthritic coils."

When he was finished, Cousins writes, Casals stood up, "far straighter and taller than when he had come into the room. He walked to the breakfast table with no trace of a shuffle, ate heartily, talked animatedly, finished the meal, and went for a walk on the beach."

What had happened was, of course, phenomenal, but a phenomenon all of us have within our grasp. It was the power of creativity, of a man at peace with what he was born to do in this world. "Creativity for Pablo Casals was the source of his own cortisone," writes Cousins. "It is doubtful whether any anti-inflammatory medicine would have been as powerful or as safe as the substances produced by the interaction of his mind and body."

The power of Calling isn't limited to the masters of art and music. It equally majestic when applied to the life of a dissatisfied registered nurse. The member of our congregation described earlier, Cheryl Pitre-Mitchell, figured she would remain a nurse forever. It was, after all, a secure job with a healthy income. A respectable career path. But it wasn't her passion. It wasn't her Calling. Then, she enrolled in the Spiritual Gifts workshop at Windsor Village, and took a written test designed to discover the answer to the question: *What are you meant to do with your life?*

It was a question no one had asked her in a long time. It got Cheryl to thinking. When Cheryl was finished with the test, her answers stretched across more than a dozen pages—showing skills in administration, leadership, and most of all, a real passion for teaching.

This woman was born to be a teacher!

She realized she had been a teacher, in some form, all her life, in every area of her existence. Even in her nursing career, Cheryl Pitre-Mitchell's passion involved the teaching aspects of the job.

"It was a revelation, like a lightbulb going off in my head," she remembers. "It was the first time I had seen my history tied to my present and my future. I began reflecting on everything I had been involved in since my youth. Even when I was in elementary school, the game I loved most was playing Teacher. Children would come from the neighborhood to play the game and I always had to be the teacher. But it wasn't just a game to me; I was dead-serious about it. Really, I felt that God had been preparing me all of my life to be a teacher. But it wasn't until I took that test that it all made sense. It gave everything I had done up to that point validation."

Cheryl Pitre-Mitchell had found her Calling, a launching pad for her new life. She became an entrepreneur, founding her own consulting business centered on her passion for teaching. Now not only does she run an extremely lucrative business educating adults in her business, she has also found an even greater joy in educating young people in our Church. She traded a steady paycheck for her passion. No longer adrift in a sea of choices, she could now make decisions based upon a central question: *Will it propel me in my Calling or leave me mired in the extraneous?* By finding the answer that had always resided deep inside of her heart—that she was born to teach—she could move forward in the knowledge that she had aligned her life with God's purpose for her. "Additionally, my financial blessings have multiplied many times over from my paycheck as a salaried employee," she says. "Best of all, I'm doing what God created me to do."

To move toward your Calling—to "follow your bliss," as

Joseph Campbell wrote—is to put yourself into the arena where real growth can begin to occur. Cheryl Pitre-Mitchell, registered nurse, would have been forever stranded in the 9-to-5; Cheryl Pitre-Mitchell, an entrepreneur/teacher who absolutely adores her work, has placed herself on the launching pad for a personal and professional blastoff. In the words of Martin Luther King, "We are prone to judge success by the index of our salaries or the size of our automobiles rather than the quality of our service and relationship to mankind." To which I'd like to add a quote from Emerson: "If you love and serve man, you cannot, by any hiding or stratagem, escape remuneration."

The rule is this: Do what you love, the money will follow. The author Marsha Sinetar discovered this firsthand. Ten years ago, she had what she calls a "great longing to change my life." She had a secure job in public education, a nice home, family and friends nearby. But deep inside, she was dissatisfied and too scared to do anything about it.

"In reality, I did not truly trust myself," she writes. "I was afraid to cross uncharted, unconventional waters to get to a more desirable place in life, afraid that—when truth be told—I would not have the requisite strength and competence to accomplish what I so dearly wanted. . . . My mind clung so desperately to the familiar."

Then, one day, was she was driving to work in Los Angeles, a random thought entered her head, "as clear a thought as if someone were speaking to me: 'Do what you love, the money will follow.'" At that moment, she *knew*: "I had to, and would, take a leap of Faith. I knew I had to, and would, step out, cut myself loose from all those things that seemed to bind me. I knew I would start doing what I most enjoyed: writing, working with industry (instead of public education), and living in the country, instead of the city."

Marsha Sinetar followed her Calling. She did what she loved, and the money did, indeed, follow. Today, she owns her own successful private practice in organizational psychology, mediation, and corporate "change management," advising some of America's top corporate executives. Her philosophies have so withstood the test of time she wrote a book about it. Its title? *Do What You Love, the Money Will Follow.*

Listen to those "random" thoughts that appear in your head; they might not be as random as they appear.

It all starts with a single question, a question I now want to pose to you: *What are you meant to do with your life?* If you don't know the answer yet, don't worry. It will eventually come, if you keep asking yourself that crucial question. That question is the first step toward finding your Calling, your mission, your dream.

After you ask yourself the first question, take the Spiritual Gifts Workshop test in the box below:

Consider the following questions. Write your answers down, being as specific as possible. Give examples. Give as much space as you need.

1. What unique gifts has God bestowed upon you?
2. Are you using those gifts or denying them?
3. What is the first step you could take to use those gifts toward your future?
4. What would it take for you to realign your life with your gifts as your guide?
5. What do you most enjoy doing? (What are your Joys?)
6. What can you do? (What are your Competencies?)
7. Do your joys and competencies add value to the lives of others?

Remember, life is made of moments. It's a slow and steady journey, not an overnight trip. Throughout your search, remain patient, always remembering that while you might not have yet found your calling your present occupation or pursuit may be preparing you to be Called. Positive steps are never wasted; consider what you're doing now as groundwork for future glory. Ask God to use your present to prepare you for your future.

The music of your Calling is all around you—if you will only take the time to listen. God can communicate to you through events, persons, or situations. Listen to God and pay attention. A personal disaster can be a wakeup call. Trust these happenings. View every moment as a gift from God. Look beyond the event at the message or wisdom it may bring. The heavens might not open. The angels might not sing. But a glimpse of blue sky in the darkness can lead you just as assuredly to God as the lightning bolt or the angel's song.

Heed your Call, no matter how simple it seems. Once you heed your call, be assured that the Holy Spirit is able to sustain and crystallize your calling.

THE SEEDS OF YOUR FUTURE
COULD BE PLANTED IN
THE FIELDS OF YOUR PAST

What lies behind us and what lies before us are small matters compared to what lies within us.

—RALPH WALDO EMERSON

"Flood is the word they use," wrote Toni Morrison of the Mississippi River's tendency to routinely flood sections where man straightened the river to make room for development. "But, in fact, it's not flooding, it's remembering. Remembering what it used to be. All water has a perfect memory and is forever trying to get back to where it was."

We, too, know instinctively who we are. All we have to do is look back and remember who and what we were before life, like the river developers, began trying to "straighten us out."

I believe one answer to *why* you were born is in the *where* of your birth, and if you examine your past you'll find signposts pointing toward your optimal future. Let me tell you about my own evolution in the hope that while reading you'll be inclined to begin searching your own past for clues to your Calling. Think of the process as something like reassembling the pieces of a jigsaw puzzle until you can recognize a pattern. I think you'll be amazed at the patterns that will appear. I know I was when I reassembled mine.

I was born on August 4, 1953, the son of a tailor shop owner and a home-economics public school teacher, in St. Elizabeth's, an all-black hospital in the Fifth Ward of Houston. I was named by a language-loving uncle who, after returning from France after the war, suggested joining my two grandparents' first names—Kirby and John—into Kirbyjon. Some might have wanted to argue that this "fancy" name seemed out of place in my neighborhood. I was brought up in Kashmere Gardens, on the border of the Fifth Ward, where one section was called "the Bloody Fifth" for its habit of hosting at least one homicide every weekend.

Although civic pride and a sense of community were quite pro-nounced, money, or the lack of it, was the common denominator in the Fifth Ward. But while we might have been lacking some ma-terial things, we never felt disadvantaged. My folks gave me a love that was warm and constant. I rode to kindergarten at Texas South-ern University with my dad and back home with my granddad, Kirby Hines, who worked as the superintendent of buildings and grounds. I rode to grade school with my mother, who taught and subsequently became a counselor at the high school across the street. On weekends I worked in my father's tailor shop, Caldwell's Tailors, at 3304 Lyons Avenue, in the heart of the Fifth Ward. On Lyons Avenue, you could see all sides of life: hotels, pool halls, taverns, dope dens, houses of prostitution, and right next door to my daddy's tailor shop, Club Matinee, a Mecca for black entertainment. On weekends, Club Matinee was rocking with the live music of the greatest names in show business, from Ray Charles to B.B. King, many of them wearing clothes made by my father.

From the beginning, I was exposed to all sides of life. I worked amid the pockets of poverty of Lyons Avenue on one hand; I experienced the soul-stirring redemption of our Church on the other hand. I lived in a neighborhood of pimps and prostitutes and hustlers and pigeon droppers on one hand and was supported by a very stable loving family on the other hand. I heard people talking about Black Power on one hand, but cried when black folk burglarized my daddy's tailor shop on the other hand. I had this strong sense of duty to my community on one hand and had my next-door neighbor break into our house twice on the other hand. I witnessed choir members who were my grandmother's contemporaries sing traditional hymns on Sundays on one hand, and on the other had Tina Turner walk into my boyhood bedroom when she came over to have dinner with my parents and kiss me goodnight on the forehead.

It was a world of good and bad, success and failure, conservative and cutting-edge. What a world of differences! What a balance! One of the dropouts who preceded me at my first junior high school was a big, rambunctious student named George Foreman, who joined the Job Corps just after being suspended for breaking a hundred or so school windows with rocks. In the Job Corps, Big George found his Calling—boxing. He earned an Olympic gold medal, turned professional, stripped Joe Frazier of the heavyweight title, and came back ten years later to become the oldest heavyweight champion in history.

The Job Corps gave Foreman an avenue, a road, a direction toward his Calling—boxing—and eventually that Calling led to his Vision: first winning the heavyweight championship of the world and later using his fame and natural magnetism in a second career as a minister. On the other hand, I watched the downward spiral of our next-door neighbor, the kid who twice burglarized our home. He could never get out of his pain long enough to find his Calling, much less a Vision for his future, and he rotted away like a piece of old fruit.

What kind of world was I living in? Where I'd be awakened by a telephone call from the burglar alarm company after another break-in at my daddy's tailor shop one night and be kissed into dreams by the queen of rock 'n' roll the next? Where I watched the demise of our next-door neighbor, the burglar, on one hand and the rise of George Foreman on the other? Where I'd hear Stokely Carmichael preaching about Black Power during the day and be awakened in the middle of the night because black folks pulled another "crash burglary," driving a car through the plate-glass window, at my daddy's store? Where I'd watch my father—without a single curse word or even apparent anger or resentment—resiliently restock his store like a patient man building a sand castle on a beach, only to have another burglary a few weeks later knock it all down once again, until every insurance company in Houston denied my dad insurance coverage?

It would be years before I would enter the seminary and read the passage in Joshua 1:8 about how God wants us to have "good success," a passage that would trigger the realization that the wealth of the world—whether spiritual, mental, or material—is meant to be enjoyed by God's children, not Satan's henchmen. But back then, the Lord had merely planted a seed; He hadn't yet led me to the garden.

From the relative calm of Kashmere Gardens, we drove to Mount Vernon Methodist in the Fifth Ward, where my parents got married and my mother's parents got married. Come rain, shine, burglary, or homicide, we sat in that church virtually every Sunday.

Thinking back now, I remember that church not as a white house high on the hill above the wreckage below, but a haven set solidly in the middle of it.

I had found my Rock, my Salvation, in my home Church. But amid the swirl of growing up, in the multitude of choices that began to cloud my vision and block my clear career path, I wasn't yet ready to accept the Church as the site of my Calling, certainly not a career Calling. But nonetheless, there it stood, a beacon, shining in the darkness.

Now, pause for a moment and consider your own childhood. Ask yourself a few central questions and write down some answers:

1. What did you truly love to do as a child?
2. What events tapped into your emotions, especially the emotion of joy?
3. Who did you most admire as a child?
4. If your life were a movie with you as the main character, is there a moment from your childhood that could be staged as an awakening?
5. When people asked, "What do you want to do when you grow up?," what was your answer?

CONSIDER YOUR NATURAL STRENGTHS— OR WEAKNESSES THAT YOU OVERCAME

When you are looking for obstacles, you cannot find opportunities.

—J. C. BELL

From the beginning, I felt that God was an equal-opportunity blesser in all areas of our existence. But the vision of Holistic Salvation was still a long way in the distance. Back then, I couldn't have spoken about Holistic Salvation even if I could have given it a name. Because I was a stutterer and a stammerer, the childhood victim of a speech impediment. Frequently, my voice just wouldn't work. I'd open my mouth and . . . it would be a verbal train wreck.

"You got to be patient when you talk with Kirbyjon," people would say. There seemed to be a short circuit between my mind and my mouth. When I got excited—and I got excited a lot—the words would tumble out in a jumble. My elementary school mates would tease me. But I kept right on talking. Although I've blocked it out of my mind, my mother tells me she took me to a speech therapist, who said I was suffering from "delayed speech," that I was "thinking faster than I was speaking."

My folks found a solution. Oh, yes, they did!

"Make the boy speak in front of people!" they exclaimed. "Let him overcome his speech impediment by speaking—public speaking!"

Think about it. When you acknowledge your weakness and offer it to God, then it can become a strength. If you stay in denial about it, then it will stick with you forever. Every time our school or Church had a Christmas or Easter program or an assembly or a prayer session, my folks would stand up and insist, "Kirbyjon'll do it!" Church programs and elementary school assemblies became my speaking venues.

Lord have mercy. I'd stand on the side of the stage at Nat Q. Henderson Elementary School, in the Fifth Ward, heart pounding, knees knocking, sweat pouring down my face, frozen with fear. My mama had given me a one-line prayer she'd gotten from *Unity* magazine to repeat for moral support. I'd repeat the line over and over and over to myself, so often before stepping out, trembling, that I'd almost forget my speech!

"God's will for me is health and harmony, and I am made whole."

There's that word again! *Whole.* Not half. I thought about this
early on, standing there before the congregation at Mount Vernon
Methodist, caught in that life of contradictions. The words repeated
themselves in my mind for so long they became ingrained within
me, a one-line mantra that would serve me someday. But back then,
I was only trying to win the battle over my mouth, and that battle, of
course, I eventually won like a boy being taught to swim by being
flung into the deep end of a swimming pool. By the time I got to
high school, that speech impediment was virtually gone.

"God's will for me is health and harmony, and I am made whole."

It was a clue, a signpost pointing to my future. I had a gift for
speaking in front of people! I would later learn that there was a
name for my gift: preaching. But I wasn't ready to recognize it,
much less follow it to where it would lead. Not yet, anyway. But
God had planted a seed. I became a young voice in my Church. I
served as steward, helping take up the money during worship service. I also made the announcements. As my voice grew stronger,
and my passion for worship deepened, the old folks began talking.
"You're going to be a preacher someday," they'd say.

I'd answer, "No way."

I was going to be a *businessman.* After all, I was extremely good at
deals. I even cut a deal with God. I was determined not to become a
bootleg preacher. If God wanted me in the ministry, then I figured
he'd *Call* me to do it. I gave God plenty of chances. The first was
when I was an undergraduate at Carleton College in Northfield,
Minnesota. I knew that Yale Divinity School offered a program for
folks who thought they'd been called to the ministry. I applied with
a little prayer to myself: "Okay, God," I said, "if you want me in the
ministry, then you'll use Yale University and get me admitted."

The representatives from Yale came out to interview me. I
made the first cut, and then, during the second round of screening,
they cut me. I got rejected. My reaction was . . . *relief!* God appar-

ently wanted me in business and I was happy to oblige. I applied and got accepted into the prestigious University of Pennsylvania Wharton School, where I earned my MBA and headed up to a job on Wall Street in New York City to make some *money*.

Your Calling Will "Call" You—
Answer with Action!

A call is only a monologue. A return call, a response, creates a dialogue.

—From *Callings*,

by Gregg Levoy

On the fourth Tuesday morning in October 1978, my calling began to manifest itself. I was sitting at my desk at Hibbard, O'Connor and Weeks, a bond-trading firm in Houston. I was poised and polished and a picture of professional perfection. I had all the fast-track credentials: that Wharton MBA and one year as a Wall Street broker and investment banker. I had just returned home to Houston three months before. It was the summer of 1978. I was a newly hired fixed-income institutional bond salesman, driving a brand-new, gray 280-Z 2+2 sports car and racing toward a six-figure income.

Those were the days when a single account could erupt like an oil well, a gusher. The lowest guys on the totem pole at that point were making $50,000 to $75,000. Six-figure incomes were the norm. One salesman at Hibbard, O'Connor was pulling in $1.2 million a year.

It was the Gold Rush era of Houston, and I was standing on the ground floor waiting for those elevator doors to open and deliver me into six-figure-dollars country. Now, let me tell ya: that was big money back then. Not many African-American males could make six serious figures in 1978—especially without wearing a sports uniform. The rest you could count on one hand: Gerald

Smith, who worked at Hibbard, O'Connor and Weeks, and a few professionals. And I was in a position, it was generally agreed, to make six figures. It was simply a matter of time.

All I had to do was not mess it up.

But there was something of that "Calling" business still stirring deep within me, a slow and steady progression, like the soft yet incessant beating of a jazz quartet's drum. It was a faint sound in the distance, but I couldn't deny that it was still there. Perhaps I began to "quality" the calling about a month before I moved to Houston, in a most unlikely place. I was at my desk on Wall Street. It was a typical 8-to-5 day, and I was a green Wharton MBA grad, freshly hired by First Boston Corporation to work in the public-finance department. Still a trainee, I was sitting at the municipal training desk when that old familiar sense of "Calling" came over me. I was not ready to go into the ministry at that point. I did not believe I was to go into the ministry at that point. But obviously, my conscious had been percolated to at least being curious about it. The old folks would say God was still planting those seeds. In retrospect, maybe they are right.

On that particular day, I called Eugene Brooks, my mother's godfather, whom I claimed as my godfather, as well. Goddaddy had given up a profitable Houston liquor store when he decided to devote his life to the Lord. He served as a deacon in the Good Hope Missionary Baptist Church in Houston, whose members included the late, great Honorable Barbara Jordan, who went on to national notice as a member of the Congressional committee that investigated Watergate.

When my godfather answered the phone that day, we exchanged the usual pleasantries and then I got down to business.

"How do you know when you're being called to the ministry?" I asked my godfather.

"You know when you stop asking and start telling," he said.

Whew. I expelled some serious oxygen. Once again, my first reaction was *relief*. I didn't feel like telling, so I figured I hadn't been Called. I filed the thought back in my "Someday" file. You know, that attic of the mind where we stack up all of our "Someday" things. Maybe, someday, I'd want to stop asking and start telling. But for the moment, I was interested mostly in selling. So six months later, I barreled back to Houston, yet one more soldier of fortune.

Since Kirbyjon was too long and cumbersome for a prospect to pronounce, much less for potential clients to spell and remember, I went by the name of K.J.

Frankly, it didn't take a Wall Street background to sell bonds. The technical part helped, but what was most important were persistence, good relational skills, and a thick skin. The really successful guys were not as strong on the technical side as they were in salesmanship and drive and determination—and most of all, cold calling. Lemme tell ya, these guys could work those phones!

"This is K.J. Caldwell, with Hibbard, O'Connor and Weeks in Houston, Texas," I'd exclaim as an opener in the countless cold calls I made every day.

In front of me was a big board filled with "inventory," the bonds I had to sell: there were municipals, SBA loans, GINNIE MAES, and FREDDIE MACS. My calling area was Ohio, Missouri, and part of New York. I had a phone book filled with the names of chief investment officers at banks, along with a profile of the bank's stock and bond portfolio.

I would do my homework, make the phone call, and attempt to pour on that charm.

"Good morning, Mr. Potential Bond Buyer, K.J. here," I'd say. "And I've got one whale of an incredible opportunity to talk with you about this morning."

More often than not, I'd get through. I became impervious to rejection. But after only three short months in that hothouse sales job, the old sense of a "Calling" soon returned, this time loud as ten thousand fans at a collegiate championship game.

Picture this scene for a moment. There I was, the proud, twenty-five-year-old Houston bond broker, blasting toward financial security, cruising down to Austin for the weekend in that 280-Z to attend The University of Texas–University of Houston grudge match with my first cousin, James "Junior" Williams. Oh, man, it was the perfect fall football day in the football capital of the world. The winner of that game would ascend to the pantheon of the Southwest Conference, the Cotton Bowl.

I wish you could have been there. The Texas heat had surrendered to the first cool breath of autumn, and Memorial Stadium was packed to the rafters. The stadium attendance had broken all previous records. Extra seats had been set up on the jogging track, and grandstands had been built in the end zone. But the fans weren't in their seats. From the first kickoff, they were on their feet. So much cheering! So much enthusiasm! So much pride! So much energy! There wasn't any sense of suffering. No hint of anyone being without. It was one endless wave, thousands of people caught up in the emotion of being a part of something.

Early the next morning, with the cheering still ringing in my ears, I drove back to Houston for the eleven o'clock Church service. Still acting as announcing clerk, I stood up in front of the congregation and made the announcements about upcoming events and need-to-know issues. Then, for some reason, I started talking about . . . that game. I wanted to share with them the energy and enthusiasm of thousands of people standing on their feet and rooting for their team. I just couldn't get the cheering out of my mind.

"Wouldn't it be wonderful if everybody would root for the Lord like they were cheering for those two football teams, particularly for UT?" I said.

And I began to cry. Now, I'm not talking about a little catch in the throat or a solitary tear sliding down a cheek. I'm talking about sobbing. I'm talking about a flat-out, full-tilt river of tears streaming down my face.

Pastor Brown came up behind me and placed a reassuring hand on my shoulder. I had stopped asking and started telling, although I didn't realize it. . . . Not yet.

"Who knows?" Pastor Brown told the congregation. "This might be your next pastor."

And the congregation said in a collective voice, "Amen."

But I still couldn't recognize it, couldn't feel it, couldn't see, hear, or know the Calling. By its very nature, a Call usually doesn't reduce itself to easy explanation. It's tantamount to explaining the inexplicable, verbalizing something that is intrinsically not verbal. There is something about a thoroughly explained Calling—at least to the full-time pastoral ministry—that would dilute the power of the Call. It's like trying to describe your first glimpse of the Grand Canyon or your first step onto the face of the moon. Words will never do it justice.

But then, the very next afternoon, my office phone rang and . . . well, it was a cold call from God. I'm serious about this. It was The Big One, as they say in earthquake verbiage or in the language of nuclear bombs and heart attacks. And it re-engineered my life.

You'll Feel It in Your Heart Before You Know It in Your Head

The next day, a Monday, at 2:00 P.M., I was sitting at my desk and the phone was ringing, not the phone on my desk, but a far deeper, more urgent ringing. How can I describe it? As I said, it certainly doesn't lend itself to easy explanation. It was a ringing that didn't make a sound, a rumble that didn't make a move, an incessant tapping on the shoulder. But when I turned around, nobody was there.

It was a *knowing*.

When you discover your Calling, you'll realize it, as instinctively as the Mississippi River knows how to return to its original course despite attempts by man to reroute it. You'll experience an inner synchronicity, an unmistakable sense of flow. Athletes call the experience being in "the zone." It's that seemingly effortless moment of physical and mental perfection, when everything is going your way. You're playing golf and you can't make a wrong drive or putt. You're running a race and you hit a stride you didn't know you were capable of hitting. You're making a speech and something clicks, and new words, deeper meanings, and richer premises burst forth. It comes from someplace deep within you.

Here are seven ways to recognize a true Calling:

CHARACTERISTICS OF A CALLING

1. Your mind (soul), spirit, and body are in sync.
2. Your synchronized mind (soul), spirit, and body are aligned with God's primary will for your life.
3. You are filled with resounding enthusiasm to begin your new journey.
4. You may not be certain which route to take, how you're going to get there, how long it's going to take, nor how much it will cost. But in spite of these unknowns, your enthusiasm does not wane.
5. You believe, sense or know that God wants you to follow the Call. Therefore, you proceed by Faith.
6. You realize that any other activity would result in a smaller or lesser contribution to self, family, community, or society at large.
7. Your enemies view your Calling as a threat, once its impact is realized.

My Calling represented the point in my life where God positioned me to create the greatest value to myself, my family, and my world. I'm not saying that prior to the Call I didn't add value. I'm saying the Calling positioned me to contribute *optimal* value, to be the best that I could be. Your Calling will combine, germinate, and package the best that God has placed within you. It represents God's best and highest use of your life. Any other use of your time would be a lesser application of your God-given personal resources. If you follow your Calling, you will eventually be able to apply everything that God has already placed within you to make a singular difference in your world. Can you imagine how awesome our communities would be if most of our citizens received and "walked out" their respective callings?

But of course it's easier said than done.

Going to work that morning, I didn't say to myself, "I'm going to quit my job and go into the ministry today." But when that moment engulfed me, it was impossible not to go with the flow. I had no idea where this Calling would lead. I didn't know anything about the seminary, about the education and other requirements it takes to go into the full-time, ordained pastoral ministry. But none of this mattered. This was not the point for questions or analysis. I was merely a passenger, riding something vastly bigger than I was. All I knew was that I was in a "zone." My mind, body, and spirit had become one, only I wasn't swinging a golf club or running a race or making a speech. I was being called by God to dedicate my life to full-time pastoral ministry.

In retrospect, I might have employed some intellect to the situation. But I was listening to some silent voice from deep within; a voice that I couldn't deny—and dared not ignore—an overwhelming feeling of *"This is it!"* It was a locomotion that overrode all logic. You just know it when it happens. At least I did. I heard a Calling so strong and fierce that it literally lifted me from my desk and sent me marching into my boss's office.

VANQUISHING THE VOICES OF DOUBT

Each of you must discover where your chance for greatness lies.
Seize that chance and let no power on earth deter you.
—CHARIOTS OF FIRE

Finding your Calling is a pivotal first step on the road to Holistic Salvation. But once you find it, then an army of "demons"—denial, self-doubt, insecurities, and a score of others—will arrive to attempt to derail or destroy your course. (We'll talk more about this in Chapter 4.) As the poet E. E. Cummings wrote, it's difficult "to be nobody-but-yourself in a world which is doing its best, night and day, to make you somebody else." To follow your Calling, Cummings wrote, "means to fight the hardest battle which any human being can fight; and never stop fighting."

This is beautifully illustrated by the Old Testament story of Jonah, the prophet described by author Gregg Levoy, in the book *Callings,* as "the patron saint of refused Callings." You remember Jonah, who was called by God to preach to the people of Nineveh. Jonah thought he was too good for the Ninevites; not only did he refuse God's call, he also booked himself on a ship sailing in the opposite direction. Not amused, God sent down a violent storm upon Jonah. Even though he was perhaps the strongest sailor on the ship, Jonah not only refused responsibility for the storm he created but went belowdecks to sleep in solitude. God's fury was swift; the storm increased in velocity. Finally, Jonah confessed his disobedience to the sailors and stressed that the only way out of the storm was to toss him overboard, which they eventually did. Jonah then landed in the belly of the whale, which three days later spewed him back onto the beach of Nineveh, where his preaching eventually converted the Ninevites. Gregg Levoy wraps up his story by quoting Arthur Kessler's book *The Act of Creation*: "The guilt of Jonah is that he clung to the trivial and tried to cultivate only his own little garden."

"If it's any consolation," writes Levoy,

so does everybody when confronted by a Calling, at least initially. Everybody, to some extent, backs away from their authenticity, settles for less, hobbles their own power, doesn't speak when spoken to in dreams. Everybody occasionally ignores the prompting of the soul and then the discontent that ensues, trying to distract themselves by counting their blessings, the reasons they ought to be happy with their lot in life, content with things as they are, things that may once have been be-alls and absolute end-alls but that lost their intoxication after five years, put them on automatic pilot after ten and became a prison after fifteen. We all have a part of us, forever incalculable and arch, that simply fears change and reacts to it with a reflexive flinch . . . and a Calling is a messenger of change, a bell that tolls for thee, and it brings on the fear that frightens away sleep. . . . In the Afghani tongue, the verb "to cling" is the same as "to die."

Following your Calling usually involves some sort of dramatic change. When you align your life with God's will, the conjunction of body, mind, and spirit, or the Calling, will become apparent. Of course, aligning your life with God's will means that you must allow God to change you, shape you, work within you. God's character, by God's very nature, never changes, never deviates. God is complete. Once you realize this—that *you* have to change, not others, and certainly not the world—you have taken your first step into a new arena of living. You have reached the gates of Holistic Salvation, where you can begin to experience true growth.

Don't expect a welcoming party to await you. Doubters and naysayers may dog you every step of the way. Satan doesn't need minions; there are plenty of human beings more than willing to do his work. I personally discovered the devious powers of doubt when I decided to give up my brokerage career to join the pastoral ministry. Naysayers rose up around me like a flock of cackling birds. When doubts and doubters surround you—and once you find your Calling, they undoubtedly will—you have to focus and press on. This may be particularly difficult when the biggest doubters are the people closest to you. In a world built on conformity, the nonconformist is destined to doubt and ridicule. As Helen Keller once wrote, "Unfortunately, there is plenty of courage among us for the abstract but not the concrete. Dreams rarely stir up much trouble. But acting on them does." Act upon your dreams and some people will undoubtedly tell you you're crazy. Take it as a sign you're heading in the right direction.

"K.J., you've gone crazy!" my boss exclaimed when I walked into his office and, without one hint of doubt in my voice, exclaimed, "I'm quitting my job and going into the ministry."

I thought he'd be happy for me. I wasn't asking; I was *telling*. But I don't think my boss really understood. My coworkers' eyebrows shot up like red flags. A few former Wall Street cohorts even cursed. I'm not going to lie: they talk pretty rough in the bond business. Soon my phone would be ringing from my associates in New York; their doubts over my decision became an unexpected occurrence. Someday, those same associates would applaud my move, but back then, it was a collective chorus of *"Have you lost it?"*

"God has called me into the ministry," I repeated to anyone who would listen.

Other people came into my boss's office trying to talk me out of leaving, including the person who was instrumental in getting me hired, Gerald Smith.

"K.J., you must be crazy!" he said. "You're doing so well. You've only been here three months and you're on the verge of becoming a real superstar in the investment-banking arena. How can you make a decision to go into the ministry?"

I was so far gone, why hold back now? "It's not a decision I made," I said. "It's something God has called me to do."

Now, I don't really recall what came next. I don't remember leaving the office, heading to my parents' home—I had been living in my old bedroom since returning home from New York—or even sitting down with my family at the dinner table. But my mother, father, grandfather, and sister all remember the dinner-table conversation like it was yesterday.

"I have something to tell you all," I began. "I quit my job."

There was absolute silence around the dinner table. It was like the food was caught in their throats. Nobody made a move for a few seconds. And then all heads swiveled toward my grandfather, Kirby Hines, who was big on making, budgeting, and saving money. His fork was suspended in the air and his mouth hung open. I'd been helping the family out, sending them on vacations, buying gifts. And now this.

"I've been called to go into the ministry," I said.

The ministry? My mother had a great-uncle and a cousin who were pastors, so we had a preconceived image of pastors' lives. They appeared to have neither any money nor much of a life outside of the Church. They lived in the parsonage adjoining the church, which was supposed to make up for the low salary, where the congregation could keep constant watch over the pastor's business. Now the successful son/grandson/brother of the Caldwell clan was headed into the gray life of no diversity, no fun, and no money!

My grandfather began firing questions, most around a central theme: *You've got years of seminary ahead. How do you expect to pay for it? How are you going to live? How are you going to support yourself?*

I had no concrete answers to my path. But I had no doubts as to my direction.

"The decision is made," I said. "I'm basically just sharing the news with you."

I couldn't be dissuaded. And then something happened that I do remember: Right after quitting my job and telling my family, I experienced the greatest sense of peace and tranquillity and inner synergy I'd ever experienced. It was absolutely overwhelming.

I had taken a major first step. I had finally taken the majestic step of Action! A long road loomed before me, full of equal parts pain and struggle, promise and growth. But one thing was certain. I was on my way to becoming whole: a perfect alignment of Divine purpose, earthly mission, and newly discovered personal desire. I completed a four-year program at the Perkins School of Theology at Southern Methodist University in two and a half years. After serving as associate pastor in Churches in Dallas and Houston, I was appointed to a much smaller Church in Southwest Houston, which had recently been renamed after the subdivision that surrounded it, Windsor Village. Prior to the calling, pastoring was not a consideration. After the call, however, it was a completely different story. I was clear about what God wanted me to do, and I wanted to answer God's calling with action.

I remember the first time I saw it, my first real appointment out of the seminary. I rounded the corner off of Heatherbrook Drive and found a quaint, yet stark one-story sanctuary. The preacher was leaving the first Sunday in June 1982, the Sunday before my arrival, leaving behind a congregation that had dwindled down to twenty-five members. When I stepped inside the sanctuary on that first Sunday, the members of congregation and even the Bishop who had appointed me probably didn't expect me, or the Church, to last for long. The Church was dying and some folks were basically content to let it die. It was, after all, caught in a "transitional neighborhood," which had turned from Caucasian to African-American. Worse still, there were already two large and booming Baptist Churches in the immediate area.

"Anyone who's willing to join a Church has already joined the other two, instead of Windsor" was the common consensus. Windsor had no choir, no music, no Sunday school. Not only was there no money, but the Church owed $54,000 to the United Methodist Church's "Room-to-Grow Program." The land adjacent to the sanctuary sported a For Sale sign—a last-ditch effort to raise funds to pay off the Church's loan and keep it in business. But this struggling Church still held fast to its most precious asset—Faith. Its twenty-five members had been praying for the Church to grow and for someone, somehow, to arrive to lead them with a new Vision for their future. But the latest in a line of pastors had departed without finding success in fulfilling the Vision.

I had found my Calling, the "Why" of my existence, my purpose in life. It was time to quit asking and start telling. We'd have to use our Faith, coupled with hard work, to revive our Church. As a congregation we'd have to develop and employ the principles of Holistic Salvation to literally save the ground beneath us or leave behind another empty lot where a house of worship had once stood.

We would have to turn the page on our destiny. We would have to make a Comeback. The devil surely meant for our little Church to die.

But God had different plans.

2

Staging a Comeback

For I know the thoughts that I think towards you, says the Lord, thoughts of peace and not of evil, to give you a future and a hope. Then you will call upon me and go and pray to me, and I will listen to you. And you will seek me and find me, when you search for me with your whole heart.

—Jeremiah 29:11–13

WE'RE ALL THE HEROES AND "SHEROES" OF OUR OWN LIFE stories. Every hero's journey involves a passage of redemption, comprising a chapter in which the hero is pulled out of the maelstrom and realigns his or her path. Redemption was such an integral process in Biblical times, the Hebrews had three different words to describe it. In this chapter, we will focus on one: the Comeback.

The place where you begin your journey to Holistic Salvation is not always pretty. The crucial thing, however, is to begin wherever you are. Just as every grand mansion begins on the scrub dirt of a construction site, most of us must begin our future on the mistake-riddled ground of our past. If your present is so desperate that you can't pull out of your circumstances long enough to find even a glimmer of hope through the chaos, much less find a Calling or Vision, you can employ the process of counted-out boxers and faded movie stars, of broken-down businesses and stalled Churches. Your future can be brighter than your past. There is always hope.

You can make a Comeback!

In athletics, Comebacks begin with a psychological process known as "humbling." Real growth can't begin until the athlete returns to Ground Zero. Just consider the growth of a young seedling as compared with a sedentary oak. It doesn't matter how humbled, low-down, desperate, or spiritually deficient you are, you can use the technology of making a Comeback to pull yourself up and rise to heights you never knew existed.

If you don't believe me, let me tell you a story about a prostitute.

Somebody reading this book is thinking, "Prostitute! Now, where's Kirbyjon Caldwell goin' with this one?"

Well, I'm going back to Windsor Village on the morning I first arrived in June 1982. I want to relate to you the same message I delivered that morning in that dying Church. Allow me to set the scene. There I was, the new preacher, rolling down Houston's South Main Street in the Volvo I'd bought after selling in my 280-Z, practically lost. I didn't even know the exact location of the little Church where I had been assigned as pastor. The estimates most gave the Church was six to eight months. Its history of declining membership and transitional pastors just made most folks predict its doors closing and its land sold for future development.

Finally, I pulled into the almost empty parking lot and looked out on the adjacent, unimproved land where, sure enough, a For Sale sign was planted. I later learned that the Church was selling the adjacent property to pay the previous pastor's salary.

I climbed out of my car and walked over to the one-story sanctuary and took a quick peek inside. I could see mottled brown walls, a piano that was probably out of tune, a Lawrence Welk–style organ, lots of doodlebugs and cobwebs, and even a few spiders. It was in need of a little "tender loving care" maintenance.

As I looked inside, my ears were still ringing with the words of all types of naysayers and negative-minded folk, who had been bombarding me with their doubts. They said to me, "*Kirbyjon, Kirbyjon, Kirbyjon, have you lost your mind? I knew you were crazy when you gave up your career on Wall Street to go into the ministry. But now I am convinced that you are insane, because you have taken this dinosaur Church. The Church has never been anything. The Church will never be anything. And furthermore, everybody who is going to join your Church has already joined the Baptist Churches around the corner. You are wasting your time!*"

But peering through that church window, I could also see some pews and a pulpit and a cross up on the wall. And I thought, "That's all I need. A cross. A place to preach. And some pews." I knew it had potential the first time I saw it. I was as green as a boxed pine; I just didn't know any better.

"So this is where we start," I said to myself, as I climbed into my robe, eager to lead my first service before my new congregation. So I began my ministry. Since there was no organist or choir, I had to serve as both preacher and song leader. My voice isn't exactly silky or smooth, but what I lack in range I make up for in enthusiasm. I walked onto the pulpit in my blue robe—a gift from my godfather—and led the congregation in a song. There were more than one hundred people: mostly friends and family and members of the Church I'd just left, in addition to the existing active congregation, which we would come to call "the Original 25."

Although the Church was in real danger of dying, that morning I felt such a spirit of high expectation and excitement that there was only one message I could preach. It was a message of God's abiding love, of His perpetual promise of Salvation, of our ability to make a Comeback, both as individuals and as a Church as a whole.

I wanted to relate to the congregation the abiding grace of God's love, just as I want to relate it to you now. I wanted them to know, first of all, that God loves everybody. Regardless of your ethnicity, citizenship, or social status, no matter how much wrong you've done or how many bad choices you've made, God loves you. His love is steadfast, indelible, unwavering.

Secondly, God loves everybody equally. God has the same amount of love for prostitutes that he has for potentates.

Thirdly, God loves everybody equally *all the time*. God's love is absolutely constant, regardless of our choices, consequences, or circumstances.

On that Sunday morning, I wanted to establish an ethos of love. Moreover, I wanted to establish Windsor Village as a Church that would reach out to folks regardless of their ethnicity or social or economic status. The Original 25 were accustomed to very conservative, older pastors—three different pastors in the past ten years—giving sermons without catchy titles. They had grown accustomed to sermons that offered quiet knowledge, good knowledge, but information without involvement. I wanted these people *involved*. I thought an eyebrow-raising story from the scriptures would prick their consciousness and stir their hearts. And from the moment I stepped onto that pulpit, I felt I was sharing words I believed the Lord wanted that congregation to hear at this time. After the song was finished, I stared down into the audience and prepared to unleash every ounce of my energy.

"Today's message is entitled Why the Prophet Married a Prostitute," I began.

If there was a collective gasp, I never heard it. Of course, there weren't enough people in the Church for any reaction to really register. But a preacher who comes in cold-turkey the first day, who stands before an audience that includes his mother, father, sister, and other relatives, and the first words out of his mouth involve a prostitute, surely must have sent more than a few eyebrows arching skyward.

"Well, it doesn't matter what he says for the first twenty minutes," my lifelong friend Skipper Lee Frazier remembers thinking from a front pew. "For the first twenty minutes, everybody's just trying to figure out what he's about."

Remembering how my seminary Christian ethics instructor explained the Book of Hosea, I "Caldwell-ized" the message of love according to Hosea, one of the Old Testament's minor prophets, who lived around 700 B.C. This was a time when the Israelites were involved in Baalism, worshiping the gods of fertility. They even had prostitutes who were "on staff," so to speak, in the Temple of Baal, and believed that having sex with these prostitutes constituted an act of worship. The point of God's message to Hosea was to demonstrate to Hosea and to the children of Israel about the lengths to which He would go to relentlessly pursue, and eventually redeem, the people of Israel in spite of their current disobedience. Arguably, God told Hosea to marry the prostitute Gomer to demonstrate something to Israel: *Just as Gomer went awhoring after other gods, so you have wandered from me in infidelity. Nonetheless, I still love you and want you back! And I am willing to pay the cost of your release.*

Now, that's redemption! But as I stood on that pulpit on that first day at Windsor Village, I would quickly realize how the cold, hard facts of the narrative would be overshadowed by the dramatics of that story every time.

"Now, Hosea was a preacher, a brilliant writer, a stern disciplinarian, a man who once said, 'Whoredom and wine and new wine take away the heart,'" I began. "But one day the Lord said to this holy man, 'Hosea, go down to the pits of prostitution and marry the prostitute, Gomer, and have children by her.'"

I snapped my head around the way Hosea must have done

when he heard God's order. *"You can't be serious, God!'* he answered. *'I'm a preacher! A man of the cloth, a man of distinction! I can't be
seen in that part of town messing around with that kind of woman!'*

"'Hosea, I didn't ask you what she is or what people would
think,' God replied. 'I said, Go and find Gomer and marry her!'

"So Hosea went out and bought Gomer out of prostitution. He
married her. But that woman didn't stay true to him for very long.

"Ooooh," I shouted in a sustained moan that shook the
Church's cobwebs. "Can't you hear that gossip rolling now: *Reverend Hosea married prostitute Gomer!* But, you know, a pig is a pig is
a pig. A prostitute is a prostitute. Not long after the wedding,
Gomer was back in the streets awhorin' and aprostitutin' all over
again.

"And the Lord to Hosea: 'Go down to the slave market, buy her
back, and have children with her.'

"*'But Lord, she's sleeping around!'* cried Hosea.

"The Lord was insistent. 'Hosea, I didn't ask you who she slept
around with! You have not always been so righteous yourself. Go
down to the slave market, pay fifteen shekels of silver, and buy her
back!'"

The message of Hosea was not lost on that congregation that
day, just as, I hope, the message of this chapter is not lost on you:
God's love for us is so strong, so indelible, so unwavering, that God
is willing to go to great depths to pick us up and deliver us. No
depth is too low for God's patience. The author of Hosea is saying
that the Israelites had become like Gomer, but God still loved them
despite their sins, just as indelibly as Hosea loved the prostitute
Gomer. They were God's chosen people; she was Hosea's chosen
wife. Just as God redeemed a prostitute out of the pit of disobedience, God is ready to step up on your behalf and pay the price for
your deliverance, freedom, liberation, and redemption right now.
God has a forgiveness and love for us that is beyond our under-

standing. It doesn't matter where we've been; the Lord is ready to give us a fresh chance to start over again.

"I like that kind of God!" I shouted to the Windsor Village congregation. "Maybe, it's just the Fifth Ward in me, but I love a God who reaches out to prostitutes, who reaches down to the places where most human beings won't even go, a God who picks lost souls up and places their feet on higher ground!"

But, I added quickly, God's grace requires our response. For every privilege there is a responsibility. Just as God loves us unconditionally, so He doesn't give us the gift of Faith for us to sit idly upon it. We are expected to use that power, that grace, toward greater good, to glorify God. Hence, consider what we call the "love triangle." The first part of this triangle is that God expects us to love ourselves and to treat ourselves accordingly, to refrain from self-abusive behavior. Second, God expects us to love one another, doing toward others as we would desire them to do toward us. In other words, if you expect to receive love, you must be willing to offer love. Planting the seeds of love will produce the fruit of love. As the Beatles sang so poetically, "And in the end, the love you take is equal to the love you make." Thirdly, God expects us to love Him. Loving God empowers and encourages us to love ourselves and others more completely. We'll discuss this in detail later in the book.

What it is important to remember now is that we must be a good and faithful steward of our bounty of blessings. To accept God's grace without action is, as the theologian Dietrich Bonhoeffer once wrote, "Cheap Grace."

"We have to accept responsibility for ourselves in order to honor the multiplicity of blessings that await us!" I said before the congregation.

And when the congregation answered, "Amen," we had, in a very real way, begun our Comeback, merely by admitting where

we were—in real trouble of closing. The next st~~~
on bringing our Church to greatness—would con~~~
But for now, the decision was a pivotal first step. ~~~
Lord was with us.

It doesn't mater what depth you have succumbe~~~ doesn't
matter where you are stuck or stalled. You can *rise*. God can take
your past and turn it into something powerful. God can transform
your mistakes of yesterday into miracles of tomorrow. God cares
more about where you're going than where you've been. God cares
more about who you can become than who you've been. Don't
ever allow the funk of your past to freeze the promise of your future! Don't let anybody or anything keep pulling you back while
you're trying to move forward. You'll never know how much potential you've got until you draw a line in the sand and look back on
yesterday and bid goodbye to your past and hello to your future.

By employing the Eight Acts of Making a Comeback, you can
stand up on the canvas of life, and no matter how battered you've
been in the past, you can now *rise*. God accepts. God reaches out.
God gives you grace no matter how far down you've fallen or how
far you've moved away from His Word. There's hope for the addict. There's hope for the shoplifter. There's hope for the anorexic,
the alcoholic, the depressed and disenfranchised. There's hope for
the workaholic. There's hope for those whose self-esteem is defined by their social status. There's hope for those who allow others to define who they are. There's hope for the unemployed, the
embezzler, the troubled marriage partner, the struggling parent.
There's hope for the entrepreneurs who have suffered repeated
failures, hope for the divorced who have slogged through years of
unfulfilling relationships. There's hope for those who define
themselves by what they do. There's hope for the hopeless!

And if there's hope for all of them, there is hope for you and
for me.

Windsor Village, we would soon learn, would be proof of that. After I finished my sermon, I invited people interested in joining Windsor Village to come to the altar. Seventeen people came forward to the altar. From that Sunday forward, an average of fourteen new members would join our Church each week for sixteen years. We had begun our Comeback.

Now it's time for you to begin yours.

1. Acknowledge where you are.

Will you overcome your consequences, or you will your consequences overcome you?

Some of us are not going to be delivered to a higher state of living, because some of us are in denial. "Denial is not a river in Egypt," says the well-worn adage; it's a dam that blocks the rivers of reality from flowing through your brain.

Our 12-step ministry at Windsor Village taught me an idiomatic expressions that defines denial:

D   Don't
E   Even
N   Know
I   I
A   Am
L   Lying (to myself)

Accepting where you are has nothing to do with where you used to be (when times were better), where you wish you were, or where your friends, based on your "self-presentation," think you are. In order to rise to the level of your ordained destiny, you must overcome the demons of denial so that you can deal with life on life's own terms.

In the story of the prophet and the prostitute, after Hosea grew to love Gomer, he became determined to lead her back to God, saying, according to the New International Version of the Bible, "I will lead her into the desert and speak tenderly to her."

The desert. Pay attention to that word as a metaphor. The Israelites were led by God through the desert into freedom. The prophets went into the desert to pray. In the Bible, the desert represents a place where people strip themselves of vanity, shedding all things that impede hearing the voice of God. In the desert, the prophets strip off their clothes, they fast, they rid themselves of the routines and processes that impede their hearing the voice of God. But there's also danger in the desert. You can hear the voice of God in the desert, but Satan is there, too. Satan tempted Jesus in the desert to turn stones into bread when he'd been fasting for forty days. Satan attempted to lure Jesus while Jesus was on a pinnacle overlooking the earth, telling him, "Everything you see will be yours." In the desert, Satan tempted Jesus with the promise of power, admonishing him to cast himself off a cliff, because surely his holy angels would rise up for deliverance. Jesus was not fooled. "Begone, Satan!" he said, words we all have to say when launching a Comeback.

We have to go into the desert of our souls before new growth can appear. You must literally go into the desert that exists within you and seek the power of God there. How do you do this? First, be willing to embark upon the search. Be willing to seek quiet, cease all routine, clear out the mind, and turn your thoughts inwardly to the deepest heart of yourself. The desert experience will either draw you closer to God or drive you farther away. It's your choice. Listen to God's wisdom when you hear it in your inner desert.

When you delve into this desert of your soul, you can begin to see your situation clearly, acknowledge it, and begin to do something about it. That can be tougher than you think, as the annals of failure are filled with examples of the eternally deluded. The spendthrift who's broke but returns to the mall like a Muslim to

Mecca. The alcoholic who is forever insisting, "But I don't drink any more than anybody else!" The entrepreneur who's counting on an "angel" to float down from heaven and bless his business if only he or she can sit and wait. The parent, spouse, or partner who repeats, "Tomorrow, tomorrow, tomorrow" like a mantra, only to discover that too many tomorrows add up a wasted lifetime.

Well, the time for waiting is over! At Windsor Village, the first act of our resuscitation was to admit that we were in danger of dying. That wolf was at our door, and if we didn't raise some funds, we would be out of business, house of God or not.

At this juncture, direction is more important than distance. You must take a first step. For the comedian Jim Carrey, whose first stand-up job was such a bust he vowed never to go on stage again, it was having the courage to climb up onto another stage and try once again. ("Failure taught me that failure is not the end unless you give up," he said.) For the boxer Rocky Balboa, the first step were those torturing early-morning runs through the streets of Philadelphia. For Windsor Village, it was assembling the Original 25 in a meeting, admitting that we were in trouble, and then taking the second step, the action, to do something about it.

You might call your first step "Convening a Meeting." It doesn't matter if that meeting is a party of one—you alone in a room with a notebook and an open mind—or a meeting with your family or loved ones. Ask yourself, as we did at our first meeting at Windsor Village, "What could be my first step?" The answer will usually be much simpler than you think. It certainly was for us.

"Get more people into the Church!" the Original 25 agreed.

"Ladies and gentlemen, you are invited to come worship with us, at the all-new Windsor Village United Methodist Church, Kirbyjon Caldwell, pastor. You're in for a joyful, Spirit-filled good time. We want to see your face in the place!"

The deep baritone voice poured out on the airwaves of KCOH-

AM, a gospel-talk-R&B station in Houston. The voice belonged to Skipper Lee Frazier, a legend of Houston entertainment, personally producing the famous Archie Bell and the Drells and setting them on their way to stardom. He calls himself my "black John the Baptist," forewarning congregations of my guest speaking engagements around Houston. In the early days, he even had placards made to post around town.

"We want to see your face in the place!"

Thanks to folks like Skipper Lee, we began seeing faces in the place. Friends invited friends. Folks living in the Windsor Village community heard the message and joined our cause. Once they entered our doors, we didn't let them down. We welcomed new members. We built a choir—which at first included my mother and sister—to help usher in the Holy Spirit. We had lively, joyous, sometimes heart-wrenching services. We became true to our mission of becoming a Church of love and redemption.

The Original 25 offered an incredible model for a Comeback, a model you can employ in your own rise. One of the most important aspects of their ability to return to glory was that they didn't resist the possibilities for change. Within each of us there is a part of our psyche that is change-resistant, perhaps even afraid of change and its by-product, success. Change can be tough. Mark Twain once said, "The only person who likes change is a wet baby." Recognize this part of your psyche and embrace change as one of the main ingredients in any Comeback.

Through it all, you must believe as we at Windsor Village believed: that there is a purpose bigger than you alone that you're moving toward. This belief will give your work a sense of joy—a joy of being a part of something that is righteous and true. We wanted our Church to be the best that it could be: something absolutely new and dynamic. To quote the movie *Field of Dreams,* we felt that if we built it, people would come.

But the first step was undeniable: We had to recognize where we were in order to move forward. Don't think that acknowledging your situation is easy. It's frequently the hardest part of many comebacks—or the chief stumbling block to making a comeback at all.

Here's a set of quick questions to ask yourself in hopes of acknowledging where you are:

1. If I were to paint an ideal "mind picture of my life," what would it look like? How does that picture compare with reality?
2. If I were to paint God's ideal picture for my life, what would it look like?
3. What are my addictions?
4. What bothers me most about myself?
5. What would I like my parents, spouse, and children to say about me when I'm dead? What would they say now?

2. Set a simple initial goal.

Maybe you saw the actor Kirk Douglas on the 1997 Academy Awards telecast. You might remember that he had recently suffered a paralyzing stroke that left him speaking with a pronounced stutter. For some it was a sad sight: the legendary actor, once the pillar of strength, brought low by age and illness, barely able to get words out of his mouth.

But to Douglas's friends and family, his appearance represented the greatest Comeback of his career, because his medical advisers had doubted that he'd ever speak again, much less on national television. His secret? Kirk Douglas was able to set a single initial goal and achieve that goal, no matter how long it took.

"The most crippling thing about a stroke is the depression," he told *The Spectator,* a London daily newspaper. "When I first had my stroke and couldn't speak, I wanted to crawl up to bed and cry. And then you get to the point where you say, 'Enough of the self-pity.' Then you get to work."

The first act was honestly assessing his situation. The second act was setting a single, simple goal. For Douglas, that goal presented itself in the form of his four-year-old granddaughter. After three months, Douglas couldn't speak as well as she could. His first goal was to speak as well as a four-year-old. One day, he said the word "transcontinental."

His granddaughter couldn't say it.

"I knew I was at least moving ahead of a four-year-old," he says.

His first goal reached, Douglas kept moving forward to bigger, tougher words, until he had resurrected his speech and resumed his life.

"Some people who have strokes just give up," he says. "And then you have people waiting on you. I try to avoid that. Someone will say to me, 'Would you like me to get you some water?' and I say, 'No. I will get it myself.' I need to feel self-sufficient, that I am able to do the simple things."

Think of it: the famous actor, who lives by his ability to speak and act, unable to speak. The famous movie star, so associated with strength, exhibiting a weakness every time he opened his mouth. Douglas is no different from you and me. Consider your own weakness, determine an initial goal, then work toward achieving that goal until it's accomplished. One goal will lead to another and another and another, providing you a virtual ladder toward your Comeback.

During our first meeting at Windsor Village, we began with the simple initial goal of getting more people into our Church. To do that we had to first determine why our numbers had dwindled down. We needed to know where our members were coming from. Then, we had to know how we could attract more from within and outside our areas. If God had joined us together as a Church, then how would God best want us to proceed into a brighter tomorrow?

This is the crucial question to ask yourself when searching for that first vital step: What is God's plan? What step could you make toward that plan? Whether you're coming back from low self-esteem, from illness, from alcoholism, from financial distress, from marital disharmony, from psychological maladies—the first step is crucial. As the folk in my home Church, Mount Vernon United Methodist, in the Fifth Ward of Houston, were fond of saying, "If you'll take that first step, God will take two." God wants to guide you. But you've got to take that first step.

3. Recognize your pain and proclaim your _want!_

When you find yourself in a spiritual freezer—loss of Faith, for example, or self-doubt—you have to process that pain, accept the responsibility for it, then proclaim to yourself and others that you want to get out. Too many folks stall on the path to rebirth because they just don't know how to Want bad enough. If you don't truly Want to become the champion of your own life, then you can forget about becoming one.

There's a world of difference between a Want and a desire. A desire is a dream that can dissolve; a true Want is a hunger that never dies. When Evander Holyfield first fought Mike Tyson on November 9, 1995, it wasn't just happenstance; it was the culmination of a fierce, long-standing Want Evander had harbored since he was seventeen. He wanted to fight Tyson so bad that fear never even entered his mind. You may say you want to gain control over your life, but if your speech remains mere language—if there is no heart-wrenching, gut-boiling, soul-starving Want attached to those words—then your desires will fade like mirages. Unfulfilled desires stack up until, one day, you find yourself wondering how in the world you arrived at the unsatisfying place where you've landed.

Consider for a moment a great American novelist, a writer of many literary masterpieces, a genius of our time. At the apex of his career, he found himself the victim of depression—but uneducated in the disease, didn't know the cause of his mental anguish. One cold December night, as his wife lay sleeping in their upstairs bedroom, this writer prepared to kill himself. He went so far as to contemplate a suicide note. He went so far as to devise ways in which he'd do the dirty deed: slicing his wrists, hanging himself from the rafters of his attic, inhaling carbon monoxide, flinging himself in front of a speeding car.

Why?

At sixty, he had long been established as a remarkable novelist. But William Styron, author of *Sophie's Choice, The Confessions of Nat Turner,* and other novels, could no longer endure his inexplicable inner turmoil and endless pain. In spite of his literary fame, he had sunk to the depths of self-loathing and despair—sunk to such a depth that the only way out this genius could devise was death! Despite a loving wife, healthy children, and loyal friends, this genius of literature could find no alternative to his malaise but suicide. Fame had left him to grovel in the gutters of depression, where Styron lost his voice, his appetite, his sleep, and finally, his desire to live. "I had not as yet chosen the mode of my departure," he tells us in his memoir, *Darkness Visible,* "but I knew that that step would come next, and soon, as inescapable as night."

On the night he planned to kill himself, Styron exemplified the power of a Want. He looked at his Martha's Vineyard living room for what he thought would be the last time. His mind reeled with scenes from his past joys in that room. "In a flood of swift recollection, I thought of all the joys the house had known," he explains in his memoir, "the children, who had rushed through its rooms, the festivals, the love and work, honestly earned slumber, the voices and the nimble commotion, the perennial tribe of cats and dogs and birds."

In that room, he found a window through which he could climb out of his situation. But the first step was rekindling the Want, the intense, visceral will to live, within himself. Realizing how his suicide would affect those whom he loved, the famous writer changed directions. The responsibility he now accepted included not only himself, but his family and friends as well. The way out was not death. The way out was life. He claimed his pain—accepted responsibility for himself—and proclaimed his Want to triumph over depression.

He immediately checked into the hospital, where, with two months of treatment, he eventually returned to the world of light. He learned that his pain had a name—clinical depression—and discovered that it also had a treatment. In claiming his pain, he found, above the throes of depression, motivation in his love for his wife and children and friends. "Although I was still shaky I knew I had emerged into light," he writes. "I felt myself no longer a husk but a body with some of the body's sweet juices stirring again."

4. Realize that God wants you to make a Comeback, but _you've_ got to act.

If belief in God were all we needed to make a Comeback, all believers would be the champions of their lives. The 55 percent of all

Americans who believe in miracles, according to Gallup and Roper polls, would employ miracles to uplift all areas of their existence. The 40 percent of all Americans who say they've heard an inner voice, a voice they believe to be God's, would be able to listen to that voice and use it to steer their lives into new levels of empowerment. The 40 percent of all Americans who admit to having experienced a spiritual phenomenon could use that experience as a guide to a Divine life. The 95 percent who say they believe in God would be able to simply employ the God force to speed their Comebacks.

The G Force, the God Force, is indeed awesome. But that alone is not going to launch your Comeback without Faith and concentrated action from you.

God wants you to be successful in all areas of your existence. God wants you free from the bondage of poverty, depression, disease, and disrepair. But God's will requires action; not just any action, but disciplined, organized Godly action. You need to set up some internal ministries.

Yes, ministries. That's what we call them in our Church. The dictionary defines a ministry as "something that serves as an agency, instrument, or means." Think of a ministry as a "tool" for personal growth, an internal office of action and organization. After we jump-started our Church, we began to take action by putting ministries in place to focus on our growing list of needs. A ministry, from a practical Church context, is simply a product or a program or even a service that meets the needs of the people and glorifies God. Just as Churches set up ministries to address their community's needs, you, too, can set up internal ministries to address and monitor your own economic, emotional, social, personal, and spiritual needs, as well as monitoring your progress. This section of this book will show you how.

The United Methodist Church had an umbrella for traditional

ministries, but we wanted to go further. We wanted to create ministries that would serve our Church in every aspect of Holistic Salvation, to help people heal their bodies, their careers, their relationships, and their financial situations, as well as their souls. If people were ready to work, why restrict the ministries to the business of the Church? Our Original 25 members included educators, health professionals, entrepreneurs, corporate leaders, administrators, and amateur musicians. Why not put their diverse talents to work? Why not create ministries for every need? Why not create ministries for every aspect of Holistic Salvation?

Whatever needs you may have, set up a ministry to help you meet it. At Windsor Village, we found no shortage of needs. There was a need to provide shelter for abused children on a temporary basis, and we came up with the Patrice House, a ministry to house abused children. There was a need for people to feel welcome when they walked into the doors of the sanctuary, so we came up with the Greeters' Ministry, placing volunteers at the front doors to smile and greet people and give them a hug, a handshake, or a high-five and say, "Welcome!" As we began to grow, there was a need to advise people where to park and how to park and how to get out of the parking lot once Church was over. Consequently, we started the Parking Lot Ministry. There was a tremendous need for support groups to deal with drug and alcohol abuse. As a result, we set up what would soon grow into a full battery of corporal drug and alcohol ministries.

Do you see the trend? Your problems won't be hard to identify. What's crucial is to set up internal ministries to deal with the problems one by one. Now, it's important at this point to "crawl before you walk." You have to set up the fundamentals. You must establish some core traditional ministries, before branching out into the cutting-edge stuff. If you have never developed a personal ministry, you don't want to haul off or even attempt to do something extraordinarily difficult. You don't want to bite off more than you can chew. You'll stand the risk of becoming discouraged, perhaps even to the point of abandoning your Comeback.

A period of self-assessment is necessary to identify which areas of your life require the greatest improvement. This will help you establish a kind of road map for your Comeback. If you are suffering from low self-esteem, you might launch a Self-Confidence Ministry. If you are an adult but still allowing your parents to control you, if you have not yet begun to embark upon what the psychologists call the "individuation process," then you need to start an Individuation Ministry, learning everything you can about the process of individuation and putting what you learn to work in your life. If your children are raising you instead of you raising your children, or if you're struggling with other parenting issues, then you need to start a Parenting Ministry. If you have a habit of spending more money than you earn, you clearly need to launch a Money Management Ministry. If you're single and find yourself unsuccessfully dating the same kind of people over and over—people with different faces but the same problematic issues—then you need to start a Self-Analysis Ministry.

You might be wrestling with an issue. Or your issue may not be a "wrestling" type of issue. Perhaps nothing is going wrong per se, but you want to improve upon your strengths. Launching personal ministries will help position you to maximize your purpose in life and heighten your self-confidence.

To begin, take out a sheet of paper and list in a column the areas of your life that you feel could stand improvement. Then, opposite each area, write the name of the ministry that will address the accompanying area. Be creative! Give your ministry names that will inspire you. Then, once you have named each ministry, answer the following questions in writing on the page beneath the ministry's name:

A. What is the purpose of this ministry? This question not only identifies the need to get something specific accomplished in your life, it also defines and sets a specific goal for the ministry. Remember: a ministry is born out of a need.

B. Whose responsibility is this problem? The only acceptable answer to this question is, of course, "Mine." Once you decide to accept responsibility for a shortfall in your life, you've taken a crucial first step. You're through assuming it's somebody else's responsibility and you've claimed it as your own. The problem may not be your fault, but it is your responsibility.

C. What are you going to do first about the situation and when will you begin? Please be specific in terms of daily work hours you'll spend, support groups you'll join, resources required, and any other possibilities that enter your mind.

D. What are the necessary resources required to address your situation? Again, be specific and thorough.

E. What resources—in time, energy, money, and sacrifice—can you personally make in order to march toward a solution?

F. Once you notice improvement, how will you maintain and follow up on your progress? There must be some accountability. How do you measure the effectiveness of what you're doing? By what checks and balances can you hold yourself accountable? Establish the systems. Write them down.

Lawrence and Hazel Jackson, members of our congregation, have proof of the power of creating internal ministries to focus concentrated action. Lawrence was laid off without warning from his Houston oil-company job. No severance pay. Not even advance word of the layoff. The cold-blooded company sent a courier to the Jackson home at 5:00 A.M. with a letter that essentially said, "Don't come to work any more. The building's locks have been changed. The company has suffered an economic downturn."

The family's income was cut by $50,000—not an easy amount when you're trying to put two teenage boys through school.

The Jacksons immediately created what could be called a Reduction in Overhead Ministry.

"First thing, we had to overcome the mental barrier," recalls Hazel Jackson. "You're accustomed to doing things when you want to do them. I kept a journal and set goals. We united as a family. We explained everything to the kids and prayed with them. We all had to work together to survive. We realized that we didn't have any control over my husband's company, so we'd just have to accept the situation. We looked at our budget. We had to cut back on all luxuries: eating out, shopping for clothes, going to the movies. We rented movies and reorganized vacations we'd planned for the year."

Fortunately, the Jacksons were a two-income family. Hazel Jackson was a partner in her own insurance sales business. And the couple had a home-based landscaping company for her husband to fall back on. Through additional advertising and asking for referrals, and help from their two sons after school and on weekends, the landscaping business increased 25 percent.

But just as they were back on track in their finances, another catastrophe struck: Hazel's insurance business partner left, and she was soon suffering under crushing overhead costs. She created what could be called a Rebuilding a Business Ministry. Once again, she took out her journal and instituted goal-setting techniques. She created a blueprint for bringing back her business and followed that blueprint. First step: Find a new location with a lesser rent. Second step: Seek new customers through telemarketing and mail. Third step: Enlist management help for reorganization. Results

came quickly. A representative from the regional office of her insurance company sent a management representative to help her set
up her new business, free of charge. Her production eventually increased by 30 percent. Since she no longer had to share her profits
with a partner, her income doubled. "The experience taught me
that we are capable of doing whatever we have to do," she says.

By concentrating focus on their problems through internal
ministries, the Jacksons were able to make a full and lasting Comeback.

5. Forgive yourself and seek healing.

If this book had a built-in choir, this is where the heavenly music
would float in. Self-forgiveness . . . it's an almost musical process,
played to the steady downbeat of exhalation. That's right—exhale.
Blow out all the oxygen from your lungs and, with it, expel from
your life all of the baggage of yesterday. Exhale. Realize that you
have to forgive yourself first for the transgressions you've made
against yourself and others. Then exhale again, and realize you are
going to have to forgive others for their transgressions against you.
Realize the energy you spend on hate and envy. Unfinished business is energy that could be used for the higher purpose of self-
improvement. So exhale and forgive. Forgive Mama and Daddy,
brother and sister, ex-husband, ex-wife, grown children, ignorant
teachers, absent friends, coworkers, business partners.

Exhale.

In his book, *Shattering the Gods Within,* David Allen reminds us
that hurt people hurt people. Confused people confuse people.
Depressed people depress people. Messed-up people mess people
up. Stupid people make people stupid. Fornicating people fornicate
people. Drunk people try to get other people drunk. Enablers enable. Forgive all these people who have, successfully or unsuccess-

fully, tried to peddle their excess baggage to you. They're all behind you now. Put them behind you. You cannot afford to allow persons and/or experiences from your past to influence your decision process today. The best form of vengeance is personal success in spite of your enemies and those who wish evil upon you.

Exhale.

And now, with a clear mind, think. One song of forgiveness isn't enough in the opera of the Comeback. Before we can bury your past, you have to make sure we recognize it for what it is. Therefore, a blanket "I forgive you" is not usually enough for real healing to begin. A deeper examination is necessary. You have to open your inner curtain and look inside at the vices and flaws and any wrongdoing you might have done, both to others and, equally important, to yourself. Once you understand how you messed up, once you understand *why* you committed acts of sinfulness, then you can begin to forgive yourself and seek the proper course for healing. When your spirit has crumbled, you can't reconstruct it until you come to terms with the forces that have knocked it down.

This is ground zero for the Comeback, a critical first step before real growth can begin. In countless stories from my congregation, self-forgiveness is pivotal: the poor parent who suddenly realizes they have been afflicting their kids with behaviors their own tortured parents afflicted upon them; the spouse whose self-loathing causes them to stray from a marriage for emotional self-esteem; the legions of mall addicts who have been led to believe that material goods can cover the holes in a soul.

6. Accept help from others.

This is the toughest part for some folks. Your mama and daddy taught you to be independent, to keep a stiff upper lip, to stand on your own two feet and not look to others for help. But I'm not talk-

ing about charity here. I'm talking about support, the kind of support that only a team, friendship, or other healthy relationship can
provide. You've got to develop a network of friends and associates, a
team whose members are rooting for your success, not your failure.
In his book *Power Living,* the body-building king Jake Steinfeld calls
these type of people Go-To people. They're people you can literally
"go to" when the chips are down or merely for support and advice.

But just as there are Go-To people, there are also Stay-Away-
From folks. As you decide to dedicate and devote yourself to making a Comeback, don't expect all your so-called friends and family
members and coworkers to be excited for you. Once you begin to
improve your life, you will begin to recognize who has your best
interests at heart.

I've discovered that it's almost like a litmus test. When you're
down and out and struggling, the folks who need their self-esteem
fed by people worse off than they are will cling to you. As you begin to make your Comeback, it's not uncommon for folks with
self-esteem problems to disconnect from you. When they choose
to disconnect from you, allow them to do so. At this point in your
journey, you cannot afford fellowship with sheep dressed in
wolves' clothing. These types of folks begin to see you as a rival.
People like success, but some do not necessarily like successful
people, particularly if they knew you "when." As these former
friends, now jealous associates, reveal themselves, do not allow
them to hamper or impede your Comeback. If you have a co-
dependent relationship with one of these so-called friends, it's not
uncommon for you to allow their lack of support to encourage you
to abandon your Comeback. So beware! Don't take your troubles
to people who will magnify them. Associate with people who have
compassion, intelligence, and virtue, people who will become
sources of strength instead of wells of weakness. You deserve associates who will be an asset to you, not a liability.

It's critical to establish a support system of people who will not only help you when you're down but will also tell you the truth about you and your situation—even when you don't want to hear it. In other words, surround yourself with enough Yes people and your life will turn into a Giant No. Yes people can literally kill you!

The Bible uses the story of David and Nathan to illustrate the power of a counselor versus the danger of a Yes man or woman. King David was feeling full of himself when he spotted Bathsheba. Immediately, he wanted to take her to his bed. But there was one problem: Bathsheba was married. All-powerful King David had an easy solution: he ordered her husband, Uriah, to be sent to the front line of battle, knowing full well the soldier would be killed. When Uriah was indeed killed in battle, David took Bathsheba for himself. Later, David's friend Nathan told the king a parable which, he hoped, would show David how he had sent a sheep to slaughter.

"Wow!" said David, not recognizing himself in the tale. "That's a wicked man. What kind of man would do a thing like that?"

"David, you are the man," said Nathan. "You did it when you had Uriah killed."

On our way to Holistic Salvation, we all need a Nathan, an ally, a competent counselor, someone who will tell us the truth about ourselves whether we want to hear it or not. When you are on the way to Holistic Salvation, what you *need* to hear always takes precedence over what you *want* to hear.

People like Nathan aren't hard to find, but for many of us—especially those with low self-esteem—these messengers are hard to accept. Some of us have the dangerous tendency to surround ourselves with people who think as we do and act as we do and tell us what we want to hear instead of what we need to hear. When you surround yourself with enablers, instead of honest counselors, you are cultivating your own primrose path to destruction, increasing the odds for Satan to lead you straight to a hellhole on earth. Many entertainers, sports stars, politicians, and other public figures are guilty of surrounding themselves with Yes people and suck-ups who would rather drink their bath water than tell them what they need to hear. Surround yourself with folks who will tell you the truth about yourself. You'll raise your standard of living to the next level.

If you're seeking a stronger marriage, a healthier relationship, a tighter grip on your career, a stronger anything, you need to create a support system. It doesn't matter whether it's one person or a dozen, find people who are not afraid to offer you honest assessment and critical analysis about who you are, what you're doing, and how what you're doing is being perceived by others.

The soul is a trilogy, comprising three distinct parts: the mind, which does the thinking; the emotions, which do the feeling; the heart, which does the believing. You need people, whether it's one or a dozen, with whom you can discuss these disparate areas of your beings. You need a counselor with whom you can discuss what you're feeling. You need a coach with whom you can discuss what you're doing, your plans of action and strategy. You need a choreographer who can tell you how what you're doing is being perceived. As we discussed, it's perfectly acceptable for the same person to address all three areas. What's important is to get someone, to take your game from the shadows and into the light where others can help you. What and how you think, believe, and feel will impact what you do. Our actions are a direct result of our paradigms for thinking, believing, and feeling.

We all need help from others, but some of us need more than the rest. If your past is riddled with half-finished projects, unfinished business, and broken dreams, find someone to help you, someone to hold you accountable. Empower somebody to help you. I know people who have struggled with adultery, so they have empowered friends to feel free to walk up to them and ask them, at any point in time, whether they are being true to their spouses. That's a system of accountability. The same could hold true for alcoholics, codependents, overeaters, workaholics, underachievers. Empower somebody to assist you in your Comeback. Find a Prayer Partner, a Spiritual Partner, an Accountability Partner, or an I Cannot Lie to You Partner.

Seeking support from a single soul will ignite a highly positive, and powerful, chain reaction: the person in crisis accepts the help of another, then the person offering the help turns to another person who can lend additional support. One hand joins another, and that hand joins still another, until a literal circle of support surrounds you.

Find a Go-To person and don't hesitate in going to them for assistance.

7. Make sure that your way is God's way.

Coming back from a crisis can be a monumental challenge. We need all the help we can get during such arduous times. Such help involves looking inward and tapping our own reservoirs of strength and determination. It also includes looking outward, seeking the support of family and friends and, of course, God. An integral aspect of making a Comeback is ensuring that the direction you choose to recover is God's way.

That can be difficult, because the devil constantly tempts us to choose his path instead. This works in many ways. Sometimes, you might think ways out of your troubles are easily accessible. If you're down and out financially, you might consider breaking the law. That's the devil's path. If you're in line for a promotion at work, you might contemplate compromising your integrity for certain favors that may improve your chances for advancement. Again, the devil's path. Such paths are detours that can lead only to

new areas of trouble—and make your life a ripe treat for Satan's
ravenous appetite. Therefore, on your Comeback trail, make sure
that your way is God's way for you.

I recently got a personal glimpse into the myriad ways we can
stray from the path. It was the day before Christmas Eve and I was
about to leave my office when the telephone rang, offering me a
perfect example of someone in dire need of self-forgiveness. Pick-
ing up the phone, I was greeted by a young woman.

"Can you tell me where I can buy a Rolex watch?" she asked.

"Excuse me?" I asked. "For a man or a woman?"

"For a man!" she replied.

"How long have you known him?" I asked.

"Six months," she said.

That knocked the air out of my lungs for a moment. "Six
months!" I said. *"And you're buying Homeboy a three- or four-thousand-
dollar gold watch?"*

We engaged in some further conversation before this tidbit of
information surfaced: the proposed recipient of the Rolex was married. I asked her if he was getting a divorce. Yes, he was, she replied,
in about a year. I asked her if he was still living with his wife.

"Yeah, but he's moving out next year," she said.

Hold on! Stop the music! Rewind!

"First of all, if you buy the brother the watch, what lie is he going to tell his wife about how he got it?" I asked.

That stopped her. That lit a lightbulb in her brain. Here's the
point, I told her. *You gotta love yourself!* Don't let Satan get one-up
on you, making you think that strapping a $4,000 hunk of gold on
some run-around is going to miraculously transform a frog into a
prince! You have to realize that there are two paths: God's and Satan's. These paths are divergent, not convergent. These paths do
not, *cannot,* cross. God's path does not delude us into thinking we
have to accept leftovers. God's path does not make us think we're

not good enough for true love, true success, true fulfillment. God's path would not involve giving a $4,000 watch to a married man on a mere promise that, closely analyzed, would be exposed as a lie.

Actions are clues. Some of them scream, "Help!" Watch what you're doing and remember: mistakes can be an effective teacher.

8. Press for results.

After setting and achieving your initial goal, it's time to create a network of goals and a system to monitor those goals and ensure constant, steady growth.

I know of no better Comeback through goal setting than the case of Superman. Yes, you heard me right. In the prime of his life, Superman broke his neck in a horseback-riding accident. The fall left him paralyzed from the neck down. Imagine waking up in the hospital, unable to move your arms and legs! Imagine lying in a hospital bed, paralyzed, after a life of leaping tall buildings in a single bound! It happened to the actor Christopher Reeve. Waking in the hospital after falling off his horse during a jump, he thought at first of giving up and surrendering to the tragedy of his paralysis. What, after all, did the future hold for him? The vegetative life of a quadriplegic. He initially considered death as a way out.

"There's nobody with this kind of injury who hasn't been there," he told *Good Housekeeping* magazine. "I remember [before the operation] saying to Dana [his wife] that maybe it wasn't worth the trouble, maybe we should just let me go."

As we all know now, Reeve didn't give up. With the support of his wife and three children, he staged an astonishing Comeback. The way he accomplished this Comeback was both incredibly simple and excruciatingly difficult: he developed a set of specific goals for himself and constantly pressed for results.

Christopher Reeve's first goal was to survive his initial operation. That goal achieved, he turned to the next: to triumph over self-pity. That goal accomplished, he turned to a third: to speak again, not at first on national television at the Academy Awards. That would come later. To set such an audacious goal in the beginning would have surely left Reeve depressed and discouraged. He set a reasonable goal: to be able to speak to his three-year-old son. That goal accomplished, he turned to a fourth: breathing exercises to enable him to remove himself from a respirator. Now, in spite of his paralysis, Reeve is working out on the bicycle. Of course, his long-term goal, no matter how great the odds are against it, is to walk again.

"As a kid, I was always competitive, and I've always responded well to a challenge," Reeve said. "If someone says, 'You've got to try twenty repetitions of this exercise,' that gives me an incentive to do thirty or forty. You have to push. If you give up once, you could become one of those people who sit and stare out the window."

Through hard work and dedication, Reeve can now breathe on his own, without the respirator, for several long, consecutive stretches of time each day. He insists he will not be chained to the respirator the rest of his life. I don't doubt that he will succeed in his goals. Why? Because he has a specific goal-setting system in place. He refuses to let any adversity stop him. He has devoted his life to pressing for results.

This is what we can learn from Superman: take one step at a time, one day at a time. He didn't attempt to do too much at first. He didn't set himself up for failure. He didn't decide to leap a tall building when a single step was a giant enough leap.

Making a Comeback is like driving in a fog. You can't see all the way down the street when it's foggy. You can just see five or eight feet at a time. But the farther you go, the farther you can see. If you just stay in the same spot waiting for the fog to lift, you'll still be in the same spot come morning. But if you'll drive five feet at a time, you'll eventually reach your destination.

Like Christopher Reeve, you can make a Comeback one act, one goal, at a time. But it will only be the beginning. Some folks called Reeve's recovery a miracle, but similar occurrences can happen to you, too!

Let me share with you a miracle from my own life. On July 26, 1990, at 12:40 A.M., my mother was declared clinically dead. While the medical team at St. Joseph's Hospital in Houston was rushing my mom from room 769 to the emergency room, I went to the phone. I called Evangelist Gussie L. Turner in Jonesboro, Arkansas (who would later become my mother-in-law, though neither of us knew this at the time), and asked her to pray for my mom's life, and to solicit the prayers of her prayer partners as well. Evangelist Turner believed in the absolute miracle-working power of God, and the Lord worked through her unswerving faith to give my mother another chance at life. According to the physicians, the probability of my mother's surviving this episode was literally 1 in 75,000. She was clinically dead for ninety minutes. But on the ninety-first minute, her vital signs returned. My mom not only survived, she thrived. Today Jean LaNell Hines Caldwell lives a very active, very fruitful life as a pillar of both our family and our Church. Coming back from the dead? Now, that's the ultimate Comeback!

Once you've made a Comeback and realigned your path with God's path, you are positioning yourself for an incredible occurrence. God's majestic grace and power will lead you, protect you, deliver you. Your life will become much more than mere existence. It will become a journey, a mission, a Faith Walk toward God's preferred future for your life. But it's absolutely essential that you seek God's primary will for your life and not be detracted by the decoy demons that will undoubtedly be thrown in your path. We'll gang-tackle those demons and Satan's numerous other tricks in Chapter 4.

Now, it's time to begin the Faith Walk, to galvanize your Want for a better life into action. Would you risk an ordinary existence for a shot at a truly extraordinary one?

I hope your answer is "Yes!" Because if it is, you're already halfway there.

You're ready to begin the Faith Walk.

To take the first step, turn the page. . . .

3

The Faith Walk

"Blessed are those who have not seen and yet have believed."
—JOHN 20:29

HE HAD BEATEN BULLETS, NAZIS, THOUSANDS OF MILES OF treacherous desert, and his own fears and insecurities. But in the movie *Indiana Jones and the Temple of Doom,* Indy is still one whale of a leap away from the Holy Grail, the cup Jesus is believed to have sipped from at the Last Supper, a goblet that, the movie promises, blesses those who drink from it with eternal life.

Of course, our hero had already come farther than the soldier who had preceded him into the cave where the Grail is resting. Recruited by the Nazis, the fool had no respect, much less belief. He bumbled his way into the cave with his sword drawn, nervously sidestepping the dead bodies that littered his path. Suddenly, spiderwebs swirled, music swelled, and—*snap!*—his sword was broken in half by some invisible force and the fool's decapitated head came rolling out of the cave like a bowling ball.

The chief-Nazi-in-charge then looked over to Indy, who is being held prisoner with his daddy, the senior Dr. Jones, played by Sean Connery.

"The Grail is mine and you're going to get it for me," the Nazi snaps, pointing a pistol.

When Indy refuses, the Nazi turns to Connery and fires a bullet into his gut.

"The healing power of the Grail is the only thing that can save your father now," the Nazi cries. "It's time to ask yourself what you believe."

Indy turns toward the cave and begins walking, reading commands from his daddy's diary, knowledge gained from a lifetime of studying about and searching for the Holy Grail.

"The penitent man is humble," he says, sidestepping the dead bodies of previous seekers in his path. "The penitent man is humble before God, kneels before God."

Suddenly, two giant circular blades slice the darkness and Indy gets the message.

"*Kneel!*" he shouts, falling to his knees as the blades narrowly miss him.

He's passed the first test. Walking farther, his next feat is to cross a cobblestone section of stones, each stone marked with a different letter.

"Only in the footsteps of the name of God will he proceed," he reads from the diary.

"In the name of God!" shouts Sean Connery from his deathbed outside the cave. "In the name of God, Jehovah!"

Indy begins walking on the steps to spell out the name of Jehovah. Only in ancient days, Jehovah is spelled Iaehova. He steps on a J first and—*boom!*—the square piece of path bearing the letter J collapses beneath him, leaving him dangling over an endless drop. Pulling himself out, he follows the letters, to the other side, only to find himself in an even more impossible situation.

He stands at the lip of an endlessly deep chasm. A doorway, presumably leading to the resting place of the Grail, awaits him on the other side. There are no limbs, no ropes, no stepping stones—just this endlessly deep canyon. Beside him on a canyon wall is a lion's head, and he remembers the words of his father: "Only in the leap from the lion's head will he prove his worth."

"Impossible," Indy says. "Nobody can jump this!"

His father's painful cries ignite an idea.

"It's a leap of Faith," says Indy to himself.

"You must believe, boy!" cries Dad from his deathbed. "You must *believe!*"

Hand to his chest, eyes to heaven, Indiana takes a deep breath, lifts a leg, and steps into the void. And there—miraculously!—he steps on solid ground. A walkway now stretches before him where, only seconds ago, there was only thin air. He walks across the chasm into the passageway leading into the resting place of the Grail.

Yes, it's only a movie, but it illustrates the concept of a Faith Walk, the next integral leg in your journey to Holistic Salvation. The concept of a leap over an endlessly deep chasm is as old as time. The movie version resembles the ancient fable of King Arthur, in which Sir Lancelot steps out on Faith across an equally bottomless pit. Once he takes the first step, an equally magical bridge appears beneath his feet.

You, too, have invisible bridges waiting to support you in crossing the seemingly bottomless chasm between your present and God's vision for your optimal future. But you'll never see bridges, much less walk across them, until you have the Faith and courage to embark upon the Faith Walk. Those who desire Holistic Salvation walk by Faith, not merely by sight. Like Indiana Jones and Sir Lancelot, you can attain the impossible, cross the uncrossable, defeat the invincible. But the first step is Faith.

"You must believe, boy!" Indiana Jones's daddy cried from his deathbed. "You must believe!"

I love that line. People marvel over the power of rocket fuel, the properties of oil and gas, the propulsion of petrochemical fuels that can fly the Concorde from New York to London in 3.5 hours or send a man to the moon over the course of a weekend. But there is an even more astonishing way of traveling, a fuel that renders gasoline obsolete and makes rocket fuel seem like useless primordial ooze.

Faith.

No engine, whether it's an airplane's or a human brain, can get off the ground without it. Without Faith, no pilot would ever climb into a cockpit. Without Faith, an astronaut would be crazy to even suit up. Without Faith, who would dare to step across a green light on a busy urban street corner, much less begin the long and arduous journey toward the hallowed gates of Holistic Salvation?

In this chapter, I'm going to tell you how to embark upon a Faith Walk, in which Faith combines with action in an incredible explosion of power. Every great achievement is the result of a Faith Walk—a one-step-at-a-time trudge toward the God-given Vision for your preferred future. Whether it's the Vision of the great explorers who crossed mountains, continents, oceans, and eventually moons, or the inventors and entrepreneurs who revolutionized twentieth-century business and industry, Faith in the power of God is a prerequisite for achieving the vision.

A Faith Walk is a journey that has the ability to rocket every aspect of your existence into brave new realms. By aligning your desire with God's preferred state for your future and by walking confidently and obediently toward that Vision, you will find the impossible becomes possible in startling ways. The first step is, of course, usually the toughest. Most Faith Walks begin in darkness: you just don't know where that road will lead you. This uncertainty, this *fear,* leads the majority to abandon their Faith Walks before even beginning them. If you have any doubt about this, a brief glimpse at the armies of easy chairs parked in front of television sets on any street will give you all the proof you need. These folks spend day after day, year after year, stalled at the starting gate.

Fear, however, can be a mere mirage. Remember: its individual letters stand for False Evidence Appearing Real. Still, fear stops many folks, and many Faith Walks. The opposite of a Faith Walk is, of course, a Death Stall, and Death Stalls begin in the same place as Faith Walks. Only the people in a Death Stall become bogged down in fear, secured by Satanic cement. This inaction invariably leads in the opposite direction of God's preferred state for your future.

So how do you begin the march toward your Vision, toward your dreams?

You have to literally step out on Faith.

THE POWER OF FAITH

When we walk to the edge of all the light we have
And take that step into darkness of the unknown,
We must believe that one of two things will happen.
There will be something solid for us to stand on
Or,
God will teach us how to fly.
—PATRICK OVERTON

Faith is a gift from God. Are you using yours or squandering it?

Some folks deny their gift of Faith. Others believe, but not enough to act upon their beliefs. Action is as important to Faith as the wind is to the sail of a ship. Like the wind, you can't see Faith. But that doesn't mean you doubt its existence. Just as a ship is propelled by wind, a life can be propelled by the power of Faith. Faith is not bound by fact or intellect.

Faith is sailing off the edge of a world that everyone else believes is flat; it's leaping from a cliff with metal wings strapped to your sides when everyone else is saying man was not meant to fly; it's creating a new TV sports network by borrowing the $8,500 start-up fee on your Visa account, then have your Vision evolve into the sports powerhouse ESPN while everyone else is saying that your idea "will never work." If you want to know the power of Faith, just ask Bill Rasmussen, who created ESPN, or Ted Turner, who publicly announced his twenty-four-hour CNN network before he knew for sure how it was going to happen.

"Faith is the substance of things hoped for and the evidence of things unseen," says the Bible.

"Faith without works is dead," reads another passage.

"Faith is believing what you know ain't so," wrote Mark Twain. To which, I would add that it's believing what you know ain't so, "at least not yet!"

Many of us pray in wishes, mired in the childlike view of God as grantor to those who pray hardest and most eloquently. But Faith is not wishing. It's way deeper than that. Faith is like alchemy, the practice of the ancient scientists who sought ways to turn base metals into gold. The alchemists never found the secret. But we have the ability to turn ordinary existence into something very close to gold by employing the Alchemy of Faith. Faith is your connection with God. If you believe enough to act without a guarantee, to believe against all logic, evidence, and advice, then you can activate the energies of Faith, the "God confidence" to realize that God has your back and you can move forward.

Faith is like a tree seedling, constantly fighting the elements for its survival. It is a battle for Faith to survive amid the constant storms that life rains down upon it. You must guard your almost childlike ability to believe like a flickering candle in a hurricane.

If your Faith has waned, perhaps you can pinpoint the stage where your Faith was not nourished. But always remember this: as it is written in the Bible, "The Kingdom of God is within you." Faith is *within* you, not *without*. No matter how many times you allow evil to extinguish your Faith, you have to choose to exercise your Faith over and over again. The devil specializes in extinguishing your Faith. That's his job! When your Faith begins to waver, you must reignite it by first fully understanding the circumstances that caused your Faith to wane.

What do you do when your Faith wavers or wanes? You decide to believe again, in spite of whatever circumstances caused your Faith to wane. There are a number of ways to "insure" your Faith against circumstances or the constant attacks of the devil that all of us face. First, feed your Faith by reading God's Word. Second, fortify your Faith by fellowshiping with folks of like-minded Faith. Third, fuel your Faith by acknowledging and celebrating the wonders and works God has accomplished in your life. Fourth, pray. Prayer increases your dependence upon God, heightens your sensitivity to God's voice, and encourages your obedience to God. Don't allow the devil to lock up your mind so that you only remember the pains of your past.

Realize that Faith begets Faith. All who have Faith ought to do good works. Those good (and faithful) works produce more faithfulness. In other words, your Faith should give birth to faithful works, whether it's creating an inner strength within yourself or within your family or community as a whole.

WALK BY FAITH

Come now! . . . Were everything clear, all would seem to you
vain. Your boredom would populate a shadowless universe with
an impassive life made up of unleavened souls. But a measure of
disquiet is a divine gift. The hope which, in your eyes, shines on a
dark threshold does not have its basis in an overly certain world.
—MARCEL PROUST,
BY WAY OF SAINTE-BEUVE

Okay, you've identified the Faith within you. Now, it's time to Walk by that Faith into the uncharted waters.

It's easier said than done. A Faith Walk involves an acceptance of things you can't prove scientifically or empirically. After all, if it can be proved scientifically, what need is there for Faith? Arguably, then, a Faith Walk is a stepping out on what God has promised you. It's believing God is going to do what God said He was going to do in the Bible—meet your needs, make provisions, heal your body, bring you joy in the midst of sorrow . . . and much more.

The pioneer psychologist Carl Jung wrote that around age thirty-five or forty, "Youthful illusions are shed, repressed childhood ideals resurface. Early interests and ambitions lose their fascination and more mature ones take their place. A person gropes toward wisdom and a search for enduring personal values begins. Either we begin a quest for meaning at midlife or we become simply an applauder of the past, an eternal adolescent, all lamentable substitutes for the illumination of the self."

In the end, we really have no other choice. To move forward, we must walk . . . but to where? Toward a place that you can only imagine with the eyes and ears of your soul. Most folks deny the guidance of the heart and soul. But then most folks never arrive at the destination of their God-given dreams. In doing so, they deny themselves of the blessings of wholeness that flow as a result of being in God's primary Will. It takes incredible trust, the trust of a child reaching up to his parent's hand. You must learn to look to God with that same brand of trust, with that kind of heart. That's what Faith is all about. It's an equation: Trust = Belief + Action. Trust puts your belief in God into action. Belief is static; trust is dynamic. Remember that childhood is where the Faith development process begins; it's where, if you've lost your Faith, you must return in your heart to retrieve it—and then move forward with maturity and determination.

In the case of our Church, we began our Faith Walk on the first day. When I stood before that dwindling congregation and delivered my first sermon about the prophet and the prostitute, we began a collective Faith Walk. We did not leap from a place of safety or security, just as you probably won't. But we began. We walked from a mostly empty Church while rumors of our imminent demise swirled around us, surrounded by seven acres of land about to go on the market in hopes of paying off my predecessor's salary.

As I said before, we had Faith, and that Faith led to action. But before we could act, we had to have a Vision. This is the prerequisite for a Faith Walk. To put it simply, a Vision can be defined, according to the author George Barna, as "God's preferred state for your future."

In previous chapters, we discussed a Calling, which is the crucible for the Vision. A Vision is the outcome, the destination, the realization of God's preferred future. If your Calling involves your career, then your Vision is a specific pinnacle of achievement. If the Calling is the path, the Vision is the destination. If you're an entrepreneur, you ought to have to have a Vision for your business. If you're the head of a household, you ought to have to have a Vision for your family. If you're a student, you ought to have to have a Vision for your educational accomplishments.

Remember this: Once you hear lots of folk saying, "No," you might have found your true path. One way a true Vision can be recognized is that everyone around you will not agree with it. By definition, a Vision *stretches* reality; it's not a quick and easy fix. It's a mountain that rises up in your line of sight, at first foreboding, seemingly impossible. But the closer you get, the more attainable it becomes—if you can persevere in the face of the negative forces that are going to rise up against you.

Consider the story of the unnamed woman in the book of Luke, who had been bleeding for twelve long years. In the ancient culture in which she lived, any woman bleeding was supposed to stay indoors. She had spent all the money she had on doctors; the medical industry had given up on her. Socially, she was viewed as a nobody; in those days, women couldn't even own property. She had been ostracized by her cohorts and exiled by her culture to stay inside for twelve years. In every area of Holistic Salvation—physically, socially, financially, educationally—she was flat broke. Busted. But she had Faith. She pressed her way until she found Jesus, who, she was convinced, could and would heal her. Jesus had so much power and she had so much Faith that when she touched the hem of his garment, her bleeding ceased and she was made whole.

No matter how depraved, devoid, or discombobulated you might be right now, you can still exercise Faith. But of course you must also walk by Faith. More often than not, that means walking against the prevailing winds or status quo.

This is where some folks literally fall off the Faith wagon. They basically refuse to give themselves *permission* to succeed. They are afraid that somebody's going to talk about them, scandalize their names. Well, let me tell you this: *They're going to talk about you anyway.* So you might as well—what?—*pursue good success!*

Until you make the decision that you don't care what evil-oriented, myopic-minded, low-or-no-vision folk say about you, you're wasting your life on them, instead of giving your life to God! If the first time someone threatens your Vision, or doubts your Vision, you're ready to turn tail and run, you're not going to get anywhere. I decided a long time ago that if I cared about what folks say, then I might as well bow down to them. You must ask yourself, Do I want to hear God say, "Well done my good and faithful servant," or do I want to hear my colleagues, my so-called friends, affirm what I'm doing? I dare you to take a God-given Vision to some human for affirmation.

If God gives you a Vision, you do not need affirmation from some human being!

1. *There are Visionaries among you.*
Listen to their wisdom.

The Bible states, "Without a Vision, people perish." I have discovered that without the right people, a Vision can perish, as well.

Once God gives you your Vision and you begin your Faith Walk, you never walk alone. Others appear to walk at your side. People with talents crucial to your cause appear. At this point during your journey, your Faith Walking will attract other Faith Walkers.

God frequently meets our needs through people.

It happened to our little Church, just as it can happen to you.

When we received our Vision for the reincarnation of Windsor Village as a powerhouse of Holistic Salvation, helping our members meet their needs in every aspect of their lives, we were joined by an army of allies to help us in our cause. Once we took the first step on our Faith Walk, a flood of extraordinary folks arrived to join us.

Some might have seen it as a coincidence. But we knew better. We knew that once a renaissance begins—either in a Church, a nation, or an individual—the right people show up to share in it.

Renaissance. That is one beautiful word! Derived from the French term for rebirth, it's been used to describe peak moments in history. In the mid-fifteenth century, a Renaissance of art flowered in Northern Italy, led by great artists like Michelangelo, Leonardo da Vinci, Raphael, and Titian. In the sixteenth century, a literary Renaissance was sparked in England, and from it came the works of Shakespeare, Sir Walter Raleigh, and Christopher Marlowe. More recently, in 1940s New York, the Harlem Renaissance produced a great confluence of African-American art, music, and letters, an amazing gathering of remarkable talent settling in the same place at once.

Whether it's great artists, musicians, or the blue-jeaned armies of the computer revolution, when like minds gather together, they can accomplish what a single mind cannot.

At Windsor Village, we discovered that a Faith Walk could produce a renaissance when a group of people begins to move toward a common Vision, a common goal.

All you have to do is ask—and walk.

"We asked God for everything we needed," remembers Pam Calip, one of the original members of our Building Committee, "and God delivered."

We needed an attorney, and one day, a man named Sherman Stimley, a Harvard-educated attorney, approached me after services and asked if there was anything he could do for the Church.

We needed an accountant. We were sent Rodney Graves, who at the time was a partner at one of the largest minority-owned accounting firms in Houston, and J. Otis Mitchell, a CPA with awesome strength and talent.

We needed an investment banker, and my old cohort from the investment banking business, Gerald Smith, offered his assistance.

Do you see the pattern? We asked and it was given.

Our ministries did not go to waste. The Parking Ministry soon had plenty to do. With an average of fifteen people joining the Church each Sunday, the parking lot was crowded with cars. We started a Greeters' Ministry, figuring that if supermarket chains can greet customers coming into their store, surely the Church can, too. People catch enough Hades from Monday to Friday. When they come to the Church, they ought to be surrounded by smiling faces and positive affirmation. Pretty soon, the Greeters'' Ministry was bustling; the Church was filled with new and expectant faces. The Music Ministry was ordering new choir robes and sheet music and filling our little church with resounding musical manna from heaven each and every Sunday.

Windsor Village was on a roll. Pretty soon, our little sanctuary

was bursting at the seams. People were literally line
aisles, searching for a seat. It was obvious to every
needed a bigger sanctuary. We had to grow merely to contain the
people who were joining us. We had a small, intimate setting
through which the Holy Spirit made a big, wall-shaking, ground-
rumbling noise. Our enthusiasm, music, ministries, and prayer began attracting dynamic folks from across Houston, some of whom
would drive an hour or more to join our worship services.

With a Vision of a new sanctuary in our minds, we began
walking by Faith, trusting that God would deliver. We started a
feasibility study to check out what it would take to build a new
sanctuary. Meanwhile, we did not wait on a new sanctuary to ac-
commodate our growth. When the first service filled up, we
started a second, then a third. It's important to blossom wherever
you're planted, even while you're waiting for something better to
come along through your faithful response. Be a good and faithful steward of what you already have, even while you're stretching
to grow.

Our Feasibility Study Committee returned with a number that
was staggering for a small Church—$2 million. Still, we didn't
close the door on the possibility. We created a finance committee to
study how to get $2 million, and the finance committee returned
with the conventional reply: you get that kind of money from bank
loans. So we began knocking on doors . . . in the middle of the
Texas oil bust, when banks were going under and once-wealthy oil-
men were seeking shelter in bankruptcy. The slamming of doors
served as a steady backbeat to our dream.

"Church financing?" the beleaguered bankers would say. "Not
interested."

We didn't know it then, but we were thinking halfway instead
of holistically. We were missing out on our fair share of blessings,
because of what we *did not know*. Knowledge is power, and if you

don't have the current knowledge, whatever your Vision, then you're probably keeping your life stranded in the familiar instead of reaching up to the fantastic.

But we had something great in our corner, something that is critical for you to instill early on in your own Faith Walk. We had what we began calling The Audacity to Believe, borrowing a phrase from Martin Luther King. That audacity, coupled with the knowledge that we couldn't do it alone, opened up the floodgates of possibility. This is the true secret of champions. They're willing to seek help. They aren't deluding themselves—or being deluded by the devil—that they know it all. They checked their egos at the door, enrolled in the vision, and decided to walk by Faith.

One of our new members, Sherman Stimley, a Harvard-educated attorney who was one of the few African-American attorneys authorized in Texas to serve as bond counsels at that time, had the perfect answer to our situation with the new sanctuary.

"What about Church bond financing?" he asked.

What about Church bond financing? Could there be a style of financing specifically designed for growth-oriented Churches? Well, yes, there was. Sherman taught us another lesson. When you embark upon your Faith Walk, the ground where you're walking is likely to have already been well tread. There are answers, resources, valuable information to be gained merely by researching, understanding, and then implementing what others have done in similar circumstances before you.

Bond financing was *perfect* for Windsor Village. While traditional financing involves payments to a bank or mortgage company, bond financing involves payments to a coalition of investors that may include individuals and institutions, even members of our own Church. The Church would pay the bond holders back through tithes and offerings over a period of fifteen years. In a sense, we were borrowing from ourselves, instead of being beholden to a bank, which, to me, is the essence of Holistic thinking—the unconventional yet empowering, instead of the conventional route.

In our case, even getting the approval to obtain bond financing—before we could secure the actual financing—was no easy task. We had to convince our Houston Board of Missions to approve our financing plan. The board, empowered by the Texas Annual Conference of the United Methodist Church to approve or deny Church financing proposals and architectural plans, was at first taken aback. A Church with big, challenging, unorthodox plans? This was something new and different! It took us three petitions on three different occasions before the board would approve our financing plan.

Finally, when the financing was secured in 1986 and work on the new sanctuary begun, we felt a surge of power, a shared knowledge that we had moved into a new economic realm. By the time we got our new sanctuary built, it was already too small. The congregation had outgrown it. Once again, we had to think creatively. We came up with a schedule of multiple worship celebrations: four services on Sundays (one at 8:00 A.M., two at 10:00 A.M., and one at 12:00 noon) and one on Saturdays (6:00 P.M.), each service with a different flavor and different appeal.

One Vision had been realized, but our Faith Walk had just begun. We kept the Faith, believing that before long another, even greater gift would arrive in our field of vision and we would be ready to walk confidently toward it.

We were not disappointed.

2. Give your Vision a name.

When you begin your Faith Walk toward your God-given Vision, you have to give your Vision a name. Because few things happen without language.

"In the beginning there was the Word," reads the Bible, "and the Word was God."

A rocket's blast requires a countdown.

A marriage begins with a spoken vow.

A journey requires a destination.

A Vision—like light, marriage, rockets, or journeys—must first be declared to be attained.

During World War II, if a soldier was encountered by the enemy, the first question would invariably be "What is your mission?" If that soldier could not state his mission immediately, he would be shot on sight. No further questions asked.

Now, that was a way to get a soldier to know where he was going! These days, a great many of us would get the bullet. We bumble through life, taking whatever we can get, accepting instead of striving, getting by instead of glorifying our lives by becoming all that we were meant to become. A mission statement is your purpose for being, your mission described in an easy-to-remember sentence, or even better, a phrase.

If you phone my sister, Dorothea Caldwell Pickens, you'd probably get her answering machine, and in her outgoing recording you'd get an anthem-like statement of her mission:

"Oooh, we're blessed that you called! Be driven to your dreams! This is Dorothea Caldwell Pickens, future million-dollar director of that awesome and powerful Multi-Million Dollar Divine Dynasty! You can if you think you can! Today is the first day of the rest of your life! Faith, focus, and follow-through! Puttin' God first! Live your dream. Have an awesome and powerful day. Leave a message at the end of the tone."

In the middle of that entrepreneurial war chant, my sister, a sales director for Mary Kay Cosmetics, illustrates the power of naming your Vision. In Dorothea's case, the Vision is to lead her sales unit to a million-dollar sales year. But she doesn't merely say, "A million." She makes it emotional, visceral, exciting. She calls her vision

"Dorothea's Divine Million-Dollar Dynasty." Each of those five words has intense meaning to her personally, so that merely voicing her mission statement gives her a real sense of empowerment.

"The name gives me something to focus on," she says. "A million dollars is too general. Be specific in the language you use. By defining what you want, what you want will be done. I truly believe that God doesn't give you a Vision without also giving you the means to make it a reality."

By giving your Vision a name, you make it real. As the adage says, "What you can imagine, you can achieve." Whether it's a business success, an athletic goal or victory, a straight-A report card, or a Million-Dollar Dynasty, naming your vision transports it from the realm of dreams into the territory of reality.

3. Set your Vision to music.

This sets the mood for the Faith Walk. If you like to exercise, you know that it's far easier to ride a stationary bike or climb a Stairmaster if you have inspirational music in your ears. The same is true for the Faith Walk. Like a human life, a worship service can be a conduit, an instrument—a piano, a horn, or a bass drum—that draws us closer to God. Few lives, and even fewer congregations, grow in absolute silence. Triumphs usually occur in loud, clanging, full-voiced symphonies of success, capped off by loud anthems and victory marches. Think of the stirring melodies from the movies with those inspirational names like "Chariots of Fire" and the inspirational theme song from the movie *Rocky II*, "Eye of the Tiger." The heroes of these films marched to their victories in blaring music, not deafening silence.

You, too, can energize your Faith Walk simply by adding some music. Music is an integral component for movement, for motivation, for growth. Just ask any sports figure training for a championship match: music jump-starts the mind and makes the muscles move! Think about it: what sports team goes onto the field without music, whether it's a theme song or a send-off from the band?

Stop here for a moment and consider your own life. Is it set to music? Is that music a riotous song of celebration or a dirge? If it's a funeral march, you have to stop the stereo in your mind and change the song! How? Just start singing. Realize the power of sound. It can dramatically change your life if you'll only let it. Pick out an empowering, spiritual and healthy song that inspires you—moves you—and makes your spirit rise. You'll be amazed by the encouragement you immediately feel surging through your mind, body, and heart. One song will lead to another, then another, until you have established an empowering new sound track for your life.

Music allows us a closer connection with God. It fuels the spirit in the same way food fuels the body. So make a joyful sound; music is a conduit through which your Faith can flow.

4. Just start walking!

We've come this far by Faith
Leaning on the Lord.

—TRADITIONAL GOSPEL HYMN

Few true Visions are delivered on silver platters with roads revealed and directions given. Faith, however, gives rise to roads and directions. Faith can become the passageway through which your Vision is revealed.

So if you haven't received the God-given Vision for your life, employ Faith.

And start walking.

Your Vision will come soon enough. But one word of warning: that Vision may not be immediately clear. Just as Columbus stumbled across America while searching for a new route to the exotic East, your Vision may be cloaked in everyday clothing.

At least that's what happened to me and Windsor Village.

5. Create a receptacle for your dreams.

Ever since she was a child, Genora Boykins *believed* . . . believed hard enough to act upon her beliefs. Her Faith took her to pinnacles she couldn't have achieved by prayer alone. A corporate attorney with a Houston industrial entity, she joined Windsor Village shortly after my arrival. But while Genora worked in the cold, hard world of decrees and depositions, she lived by Faith. Even when she and her husband began building their new house—before their old one had been sold—she employed Faith against the prevailing wisdom of a then recession-plagued Houston real estate market, never doubting. "I just knew the Lord would provide a way," she says.

And the Lord did. Her old house sold before her new house was completed. Once again, her Faith saw her through.

When Genora Boykins walked into Windsor Village, she was seeking a way to serve. Eventually, she came to serve in precisely the way we most needed. It was extraordinary timing, but that's the way God works. People have probably walked into your life seeking to serve. But you might not have recognized them as potential allies in your cause. All of us are literally surrounded by potential support, but we must step out of our own shadows to find it, much less receive it.

Genora joined the Greeter's Ministry, a ministry that primarily consumes time only on Sundays. Perfect for a busy corporate attorney. But then one day she heard about our Legal Ministry, which was set up primarily to offer legal advice and educate our members in the world of law. Genora began talking with the ministry's coordinator, who was leaving to take care of her two small children. She asked Genora to take over the ministry, and Genora graciously accepted.

I was interested in her thoughts about the potential of the Legal Ministry and asked her to meet me one morning for breakfast in southwest Houston. After all, if Holistic Salvation involves enlisting the power of God in every aspect of our existence, what truly sanctified soul, or congregation, can exist today without a lawyer? We discussed a few potential projects and came to the same decision: Our first step would be to create a community development corporation (a CDC), a nonprofit corporation under which Churches and other nonprofit entities had developed housing and other projects. In our case, we weren't thinking about subdivisions. Not yet. But a small amount of property had been donated to the Church, and a CDC could help us develop and eventually sell the property. I asked Genora if she would set up the CDC.

Genora said she'd "pray on it," which you might think is a strange way for an attorney to make a decision. But for Genora Boykins, it's a perfectly effective way of decision making.

"If I have a peaceful night's sleep, if I don't toss and turn, if I don't feel any trouble in my spirit, then I know it's right," she says. "The way the Lord speaks to me is by giving me a sense of inner peace."

Genora called the next morning. She'd slept well. She would set up the CDC.

We called it the Pyramid Community Development Corporation, the name representing a building in ancient Egypt, which, we felt, was a good representative of what we were trying to do: build something that would last longer than ourselves. In retrospect, in establishing our own CDC we were doing something incredibly vital to the future development of our Church, something that you also must do to lay the groundwork for your own optimal future.

You have to create a receptacle for your Vision, even if that Vision has not yet become apparent.

Of course, we didn't know any of this back then. We soon had our own CDC, but aside from the small amount of property we'd been given, nothing to put into it. Something incredible happened, though, when we started that CDC. We became qualified in a field where we'd been unqualified before. We had opened ourselves up to receive. We had created a receptacle to hold and manage whatever blessings appeared.

What could serve as a receptacle in your life—an education? a loving home? a stable psychological foundation?—to hold your Vision once it appears?

RULES FOR THE ROAD

A Faith Walk is further propelled by good stewardship, which essentially means being a good steward, a good manager, of whatever God has given you: talents, gifts, spiritual gifts, properties, and finances. Let's study a few principles of good stewardship:

The Who's-in-Charge Principle. God is the owner; we are the manager. Once you come to understand that God is in charge of your life, you'll have a whole new perspective on things. Once the who's-in-charge principle is resolved, everything else becomes matter-of-fact. You serve; God gives.

The Give-and-Grow Principle. As we learn how to give and sow seed in God's kingdom, we grow in abundance. You cannot give back to God without growing spiritually, relationally, financially. When you give, God gives back to you. When God blessed you, He did not have you in mind. God expects the blessings to flow through you to those who are around you. You reap what you sow.

Identify Your Spiritual Gifts. When you practice stewardship, you're able to find your spiritual gifts. I cannot pray as long and as effortlessly as Barbara Hicks does. My teaching gift is not as strong as my wife Suzette's. I can't sing like our Minister of Music, Hanq Neal. And I don't worry about the gifts that I don't have and others do. I just want to do what God is calling me to do. Sometimes we sit on our spiritual gifts because we can't do something as well as somebody else. Nobody's asking you to do something the way somebody else does it. There's nobody here like *you!* Do what God is calling *you* to do! And do that to your very best.

Increase Your Faith. When you discover your spiritual gifts and practice them, your own Faith increases. If you want to grow in your Faith, practice it. In East Texas, there are some pigs that eat and eat and eat and never grow. That's the definition of a runt. The world is full of spiritual runts. People who come to Church, who come to Bible study, who suck up all the meat and the milk but never grow.

Become Spiritually Sensitive. God wants you to have an advantage over the children of darkness. You are a child of light, who's led by God's Spirit, and God wants to show you things before they happen. When you're spiritually sensitive, you can hear God in other places than your ears. No matter how much racism, narcissism, sexism, or any other kind of "ism" is operating against you, when you are grounded in God and you've been a good and faithful steward of what God has given you and Who God is, the very gates of hell cannot prevail against you.

Be a Blessing. God's blessing of you is dependent on your willingness to be a blessing. After all, why should God trust you with more when you haven't proved to be a good and faithful steward of what you have right now? If you're a cantankerous single person, why should the Lord bless you with a spouse? If you're an unproductive employee, why should the Lord bless you with a raise? If you can't show up on time for the 9-to-5 job you have now, why should God promote you to manager? We should want to be a blessing and not just receive a blessing.

Remember Your Indebtedness. We're not talking strictly about financial debts, but a twofold indebtedness. Remember, you're indebted to both God and your previous generation. Your parents and grandparents may have made less money in six months than you make in two months. But they managed to lend you money. They prayed for you when you didn't know what prayer was. They sacrificed to get you through college. Honor them, just as you honor God.

VISION: YOUR SIGN FROM ABOVE

Vision. . . . It reaches beyond the thing that is, into the conception of what can be. Imagination gives you the picture. Vision gives you the impulse to make the picture your own.
—ROBERT COLLIER

It arrived in the spring of 1992, a mountaintop at first shrouded in clouds, then startling in its size and majesty. It was so big, so vast, so impossible that we didn't even recognize its potential at first, much less think such an immense project could be meant for us. But when the doubts began arising in our minds, and the naysayers began carping negatives, we took it as a sign that we might be on to something.

I had seen it countless times on my way to the Church. Coming off the 610 Freeway, heading south toward Windsor Village, you couldn't miss the big, asbestos-choked vacant Kmart. It was a 104,000-square-foot reminder that boomtowns don't always last, one more sign of Houston's economic downturn in the late eighties.

This abandoned building was the site of a bona fide Vision. But I couldn't see it at first. It didn't ignite neon signs in my mind or even whisper, "Slow down, Kirbyjon, there's an incredible Vision in the middle of your windshield!" Burning bushes, sadly, never really blaze until you pour the gasoline of your intellect, and your Faith, upon them.

But once you begin talking to God, and start walking by Faith, God begins communicating. Sometimes His answers arrive in a language far more majestic than mere words. God often speaks in actions, blessings, and words, through humans, and an infinite number of other forms. These actions, blessings, and words will probably encourage you, ask you to step up and do something to claim the prize that God has in store for you.

That's what happened to our Church.

"Can you think of anybody in the community that might have a use for this place?"

It was July 1992, and Buster Friedman, president of United Equities, the real estate consulting firm for Fiesta, Inc., which operates mega-supermarkets across Texas, was on the telephone. The "place" that he was referring to was a vacant, rat-infested 104,000-square-foot Kmart store. Fiesta, whose supermarket sat next-door to the Kmart, owned the land and was eager to lease it. To most people, it was an eyesore.

In retrospect, I should have seen the promise that the vacant building held.

For ten years I had been preaching about Holistic Salvation, about a God that blesses every aspect of our existence, and now God was placing a bona fide Vision in our path. As I said, at first I was too blind to recognize it. But God found a way to show it to me and our Church.

The real estate folks have a generic term for the strip malls popular in the Southwest, the ubiquitous shopping centers anchored by a few big, usually national chains, which are surrounded in the strip by smaller, usually local merchants. They call these collections of buildings "power centers." When Donald Bonham, the chairman of Fiesta, Inc., and Buster Friedman asked me if I had any ideas for rejuvenating the site, I didn't immediately have any ideas. But I didn't say, "No." I didn't close the door. I said, "Give me a few days to think about it and pray on it."

Remember this when potentially empowering situations seem to literally fall into your lap: *The shoe does not tell the foot how fast to grow*. Which is to say, once God has given you His preferred Vision, then it's very important for your mission statement and your structure and your systems and your principles and practices to line up and bow down to the Vision. The Vision and the mission should never have to bow down to the structure.

When you're growing, your shoe does not tell your foot how fast to grow. Remember when your foot was growing? What did you do when you outgrew a shoe? You got another shoe. You didn't try to stuff your bigger foot into that old small shoe. Every living organism grows. Things that grow naturally stretch the status quo. Real growth always involves change.

So when opportunities seem to fall in your lap, don't toss them out because you do not yet have the "structure" to support them. Things happen for reasons. Many gifts from God wind up in the garbage merely because the receiver is unable to see the gift for what it is or what it can become. Always try to recognize the reason behind the happening. And most important, remember this: When in doubt, ask for enlightened advice.

I took that all-important question "Can you think of anybody who might have a use for this place?" to some very enlightened allies: our regular Bible-study meeting at Windsor Village. Almost reflexively, several people immediately replied, *"What about us?"* Now, that's a healthy response! They recognized a Vision in the vacant storefronts. They didn't see the decay of the vacant shopping center but the promise of what it *could* become. Their focus was on one four-letter word: *jobs.* If we could somehow develop the vacant power center ourselves, what kind of jobs could we offer our congregation and our community?

What about us?

Think about it. *What about you?* When an opportunity arises— when something is practically thrown in your lap—what about you? The old folks say, "Don't look a gift horse in the mouth." You might mistake diamonds for decay.

As I've said, I had been endlessly preaching about Holistic Salvation, about a God who stands ever ready to grant fulfillment in every aspect of our existence. But our members had to go outside the Church to find fulfillment in many important areas of their lives. We wanted our people employed, but we didn't have any jobs to offer. We wanted our congregation uplifted, but what were we doing to salvage the recently empty shopping centers and abandoned storefronts plagued by the eighties oil bust? We wanted the children in our congregation educated, but we didn't have our own school. We wanted our community economically fulfilled, but we couldn't even cash their checks, much less offer them investment opportunities. Our entire community did not even have one bank branch!

I didn't realize it then, but now I can see that we were a classic case of "left-brain thinking," and were thus missing out on one-half of the possibilities that "whole-brain thinking"—or Holistic Thinking—can bring. The brain is, of course, one of God's most awesome creations, a universe unto itself in which an estimated one million chemicals and ten million individual nerve cells are constantly reacting. It's been proved that the brain, which is physically divided into two halves, and separated by a bridge known as the corpus callosum, divides thought dominance in most humans into one of the halves.

All of us use both sides of our brains, but most of us rely on
one half more than the other. Left-brain thinkers are strong in language, logic, reason, and computation, but weak on the right-brain,
creative aspects that could allow them to apply their intellect in
new and creative ways. Right-brain thinkers—whose strengths are
imagination, rhythm, musical appreciation, images, and pictures—
can be highly creative and intelligent. But they can be disorganized
when it comes to logic, reason, and computation, all of which lie in
the territory of the left brain.

Maybe you're a classic left-brain thinker, but without the right-
brain "logic," you may have jettisoned creativity in your life. On
the flip side, perhaps you're so right-brain-oriented, you've become fogged in by your own creative nature and are missing the
propulsion that logic and linearity could bring to your life.

If you recognize yourself as a primarily left- or right-brain
thinker, seek out more information on the subject. Plenty exists.
But the most important thing is to realize that God graced you with
a *whole* brain, not a half. You can jump-start the less utilized half of
your brain merely by realizing that you were given a whole brain to
use both halves.

Then allow the Lord to bless you by seeing your Faith Walk
through His eyes and not just your own. That's when the transformation *really* occurs. Once you entrust your Faith Walk to God,
then you can truly experience whole-brain thinking. In pursuing
God's primary will for your life in general and your projects in particular, the Lord will provide you with whatever is missing. In the
case of our Church, whenever we found ourselves looking at a project in some of our typically left-brain ways, God stepped in and
gave us the right-brain perspective.

Realize that Satan is a master of deceit, a magician of chaos.
One of his favorite and most effective cons is to convince us that
we suffer from shortcomings and slights that block our path to

growth and rejuvenation. That we're not good enough, smart enough, young enough, old enough, tough enough, left- or right-brain enough . . . Was Satan trying to convince me and my Church to remain mired in the status quo belief that Churches are meant for prayer and not social development? He was certainly doing his best to do so. But the mere fact that our Vision was *against* the common wisdom was a sign that it was the real thing. Real Visions usually encounter "Why-you-wanna-do-that?" people. It's like gravity. The conventional world will always attempt to keep the striver's feet firmly planted on the ground. But you have to first recognize, and then resist, these evil forces. You have to say, as Israeli prime minister Golda Meir once stated, paraphrasing Hillel, "If not me, then who? If not now, then when?"

But I must admit that I, too, was gripped by conventional thinking—until I took a trip to Jonesboro, Arkansas, for a family reunion in 1992. During my visit, I paid a visit to the local Wal-Mart, and God gave me a Vision right there between the housewares and the cleaning supplies. There I was, standing in the middle of that smorgasbord of commerce, when a Vision reached down and knocked me off my feet with its power and clarity. If a commercial store could offer "one-stop shopping," with everything under one roof, why couldn't a Church? Why couldn't we become the Wal-Mart of Holistic Salvation, offering a smorgasbord of services—medical, financial, educational, emotional—to our community?

If every step of our lives eventually serves God's Vision for our life, then perhaps my degree from the Wharton School of Business and my years in the investment banking business had been part of God's purpose and plan. It certainly seemed that way. Windsor Village was going into the business of empowerment.

We were going to step up to the plate and claim what was ours. We had the audacity to believe—the Faith—that we were entitled to Holistic Salvation, fulfillment in every aspect of our existence. Then and only then could we begin our Faith Walk toward achieving our Vision.

We began new discussions with Fiesta Mart, with important new emphasis. We shifted the vague to the specific. We had some ideas about how to revitalize the vacant building, and that idea could be stated in a three-word sentence: *"What about us?"*

GOD'S GOT YOUR BACK

"Hey, what about us?"

This was the question our Pyramid CDC committee, consisting of four Church members and myself, began asking, first once and then a hundred times.

We could use that empty asbestos-filled building. In a nation where more than a hundred folks get murdered daily, where every day thousands of our young women become pregnant before they are ready, where people use folk and love things, what Church couldn't use a shelter from the escalating storm? We asked ourselves the single most important thing to consider when presented with a possible Vision: If God meant this for us, what would He have us do with it?

The answer was immediately clear: God would have us use that building for Holistic Salvation, to serve our congregation and our community in every area of our existence: financially, emotionally, educationally, medically, and physically. Ideas bubbled forth from our group in a deluge: We'd have our own bank, school, health clinic, college branch, social service agencies, meeting rooms, and much, much more. We wouldn't be an island, however; we'd be a bridge to our community and to the outside world. The building would empower us in infinite ways. We would finally own, not rent; employ, not merely be employed; we'd be the landlord, not the lessee; we'd become our own bosses, instead of remaining employees enjoined by conventional jobs, leases, and loan payments.

We would follow a passage from Isaiah 61 in the Bible, "They shall rebuild the old ruins, they shall raise up the former desolations, and they shall repair the ruined cities."

We had found our mission statement. Soon, we gave our Vision a name. All we had to do was capitalize it: the power center became The Power Center.

We knew we were on to something incredible, something akin to what film director Steven Spielberg must feel when he finds a great story. How does he know it's great? "When I read, I count the goosebumps," he once said.

We had *serious* goosebumps.

If we could dream it, we could do it. And you can, too. As we discussed, God won't give you a Vision without also giving you the means to fulfill it. That doesn't mean it's going to be easy. You're going to have to walk. But once you do, your road will eventually become clear.

Our committee of five was not a collection of moguls. We were absolutely everyday people, each equipped with his or her own special talents: Al Scarborough, the human resources specialist; Genora Boykins, the attorney; J. Otis Mitchell, the CPA; Maude Collins, the local homemaker; and me. Tina Moore served as the executive director of our Pyramid Community Development Corporation.

What separated us from the pack is what also has the ability to separate you from the masses: our audacity to believe. That belief, we soon discovered, was half the battle. We knew that God had our back, and with that knowledge, we could forget the past and move forward into the future.

"God's got my back." That's a line I keep hearing from members of our congregation. I hear it so often, I think of it almost as a motto for the Faith Walks that the people who say it are usually taking.

I think of young people like Andrea Sadbury, a sixteen-year-old Houston high school student, who valiantly tried to keep her parents together during a particularly rough period in their marriage. Andrea tried so hard at "saving the world," as she puts it, her grade-point average plummeted in the process. Only when she learned to trust God to resolve the situation and step out onto her own Faith Walk did Andrea find peace. Her grades returned to honor-student status and her parents eventually reunited.

I think of Lemuel McNeil, a young home builder, who placed his résumé on our altar one day, asking God to bless his career. Then, he grabbed that résumé and began a Faith Walk to daily interviews, hopscotching through three different firms over the last ten years, first doubling, then tripling his salary and status in the firms before eventually landing what he considers his dream job. "You have to believe," Lemuel says.

I think of Lynn Gooden, a young elementary school teacher, who says she's been on a Faith Walk since she was sixteen. "I pray for something and—*bam!*—it eventually happens," she says. But that *bam!* never happens while Lynn's sitting in some easy chair, flipping channels on a TV set. This woman walks! She walked out of a tortured marriage to a crack-addicted husband to become an amateur gospel singer. She walked from praying for a home of her own to realizing that Vision. "Every time I walk on Faith, it's like the windows of heaven open up," she says.

But most of all I think of our congregation in October 1992, when we were able to tell them that Donald Bonham and Fiesta Mart had agreed to donate the vacant Kmart building and 25 acres of land to our community on or after March 31, 1993. Mr. Bonham's generosity, community sensitivity, and civic commitment were astounding and should be vigorously applauded.

We had our Vision spread out before us, and the Holy Spirit listened to our Vision.

Now, we had to walk toward creating that Vision in that empty building. It was a long and arduous journey. But in the beginning we followed a few simple, yet critical guidelines. In reading about our Faith Walk over the next few pages, please substitute your own Vision and focus on it. I hope you'll be able to see how a Faith Walk can lead you into the real world of achieving your dreams.

We discovered that most Faith Walks essentially have four main legs:

1. *Faith.* This is the audacity to put God's promise into action. God's Vision for your preferred future is going to be greater than your present situation . . . or what kind of Vision would it be? Admit in the beginning that you're going to need help from others. This admission opens your life up to receiving help, advice, information, and assistance. There are talented people eager to help you. All you have to do is ask and accept. Never consider yourself above criticism, beneath redemption, or beyond hope. Allow yourself to receive help! Know-it-alls will soon lose it all.

2. *Focus.* Your mission statement is your purpose for being. It is the present tense of your "Vision statement," which is future-oriented. Once your Vision becomes clear, construct a mission statement and give your Vision a name. Then, keep that Vision always in mind, never allowing the "decoy demons" to steer you off track. Remember Peter in the Bible, walking on the stormy sea of Galilee, after having being beckoned by Jesus to walk toward him? As long as Peter kept his eyes on Jesus, the Author of his Faith, he was able to walk on the water just fine. But as soon as he took his eye off Jesus and began to focus on the elements, he began to sink. You've got to keep your eyes on the prize—on the Vision—and not be distracted by the elements. In our case, we had to remember that our Vision wasn't merely about building buildings or raising money to build buildings. Our Vision

was about creating a Power Center that praises God and empowers people. We kept our mission statement forever foremost in our minds, using it on letterheads, on signs, and in conversation, and that kept us afloat in even the rockiest moments. Post your own mission statement in a place where you will see it daily, and don't be distracted as you move toward your Vision.

3. *Action.* This is, of course, the "Walk" of the Faith Walk, the toughest part for some folks. This is where the rubber meets the road. When you step out into that void, step with the confidence that when you take the first step, God will take two steps behind you. That's God's majesty at work. He doesn't always show you the entire journey before it begins. Sometimes He shows you just enough to keep you going, growing, moving. If we had known that our Power Center would take eighteen months instead of eight months to complete, if we had known it would take $5 million instead of our estimated $2.8 million, if we had been shown all of the close calls and narrow misses that would litter our path, we might not have taken even the first step. We might have been paralyzed at the starting gate. We learned that you walk by Faith the way you would eat an elephant: one bite, one step, at a time. God will show you just enough to keep you moving forward—if you can just take that first step.

4. *Prayer and Praise.* This is the continuous power of Faith, the constant glory that you give to God. Prayer is the most underutilized asset in America. We started our prayer ministry at Windsor Village thirteen years ago. It's proved to be such a crucial component of our Church that I recently asked my wife, Suzette, to head it up. In the next few chapters of this book, you will see how prayer lifted our Church and congregation to heights of which we wouldn't have dared dream. But we discovered that when you pray, God will direct your path.

Finally, once you embark upon a Faith Walk, be sure to relish the journey instead of constantly focusing on the destination. When God gives you the glory of a Vision, employ your Faith and begin the walk, appreciating the wonders that will soon stretch out before you.

In the case of our Church, we began our walk. Our Faith was strong, our Vision in sight.

Now, only the devil could trip us up—if we allowed him to do so! And sure enough, he began to try.

4

Whuppin' the Devil

Be sober, be vigilant; because your adversary, the Devil, walks about like a roaring lion, seeking whom he may devour.
—1 PETER 5:8

The biggest trick the devil has played on us is that he convinces us he does not exist.

—AL PACINO IN
THE DEVIL'S ADVOCATE

YOU DON'T BELIEVE IN THE DEVIL? YOU THINK HE'S SOME cartoon character or Biblical fairy tale? A demon confined to the imagination of devil worshipers and overheated ministers? I'm here to tell you that the devil exists—not as some simplistic, one-dimensional character, but as an amazingly nimble, informed, high-tech spirit that has the ability to morph and mutate, like a deadly disease, into infinite realities and invade every aspect of your existence. Talk about a terrorist! We're dealing with the nuclear bomb of all evils, a grenade detonating constantly and with no signs of cessation.

Yes, the devil exists! And he's out to get you! The Bible reminds us that the devil is on what we'll call a "s.k.a.d." mission: he wants to steal, kill, and destroy.

On a fairly regular basis, I like to preach one of those fundamental, down-home, slam-dunk sermons on how to whup Satan. Not whip, but *whup*. There is a *big* difference between a whipping and a whuppin'. I used to catch whippings, but every now and then I'd catch a whuppin'. It's a whuppin' when you're told to pick your own switch from the clump of hedges and trees in the backyard—and the first switch you bring in is always too small. Your mama or your daddy will say, "Go get one that's a little bit more deserving for what you've done here." They're not satisfied until you find one that appears—through the eyes of intimidation—to be roughly the size of a cane fishing pole. And then your mama or your daddy starts not whipping you but *whuppin'* you. You know you're getting a whuppin' when they preach while they're tanning your hide. Another characteristic of a whuppin', not merely a whipping, is when Mama says, "I'm whuppin' you now so the cops will not have to whup you later."

Let me tell you how to *whup* Satan—before he whups the tar out of you.

WHO IS SATAN?

"How are you fallen from heaven, day star, son of the dawn! How are you fallen to earth, conqueror of nations! You said in your heart, 'I will ascend to heaven, above the stars of God; I will set my throne on high. . . .' But you are brought down to darkness, to the depths of the pit."

—ISAIAH 14:12–15

Before you can whup the devil, you have to find him, which is not always easy. For we're dealing with the most sinister criminal in creation, a serial killer with more aliases, disguises, and alibis than all the master crooks of the world combined.

When most folks consider the devil, they think about some cartoonish creature dressed up in a red jumpsuit, with pointy ears, a lunatic leer, and a pitchfork. If you are looking for this particular manifestation, you will never encounter the devil except on your front stoop on Halloween night. The real devil is far wilier than to restrict himself to a single silly costume. The real devil is the absolute *master* of masquerade. He is not only extraordinarily devious and deceptive, but the eternal enemy of God. The devil is, in a word, God's foremost adversary. And since he can't get to God, he takes delight in destroying God's creation—humankind. If you don't believe in Satan, then he's already winning his war to control you, and believe me, Satan is waging a constant war against you, whether you acknowledge it or not.

Who is this ultimate agent of destruction? One of the best definitions comes from John A. Sanford's book *Evil: The Shadow Side of Reality*. Sanford writes that the word *Satan* is a carryover from the Hebrew word that means "a being that hinders free, forward movement." The word *devil* is derived from the Greek word, *diabolos,* which, as a verb, literally means "to throw across." As a noun, *diabolos* is translated as an accuser or adversary, which corresponds closely to the traditional meaning of the word *Satan.*

In the Gospel, Satan is held responsible for numerous ailments and afflictions, sicknesses and diseases, everything from plagues to singular maladies, like a woman who for eighteen years could not stand erect. Satan appears in the Gospel as the spirit opposed to God, who throws every obstacle in the path of humankind, perpetually attempting to divert our quest for health, wholeness, and completeness. Additionally, Satan also strives to turn you from God, yourself, and your neighbor by encouraging rebellion, disloyalty, and hatred.

The Greek word for obstacle is *skandolon,* which means "stumbling block." At the risk of oversimplifying an extremely complicated issue, Satan is in the business of throwing obstacles, hindering free and forward movement, and creating stumbling blocks.

I tell you these stories to show you how Satan will use lies, illusions, rumors, and anything else he can muster to "throw across" your path of Divine direction, deliverance, and determination. Satan's involvement should be expected and, frankly, anticipated. The question is not whether he will intervene in a path or a process of godliness, but how and when. Being able to anticipate Satan's move and timing increases the possibility of winning your war against him.

Pay special attention to how Satan tempts you personally. Note how he strives to throw obstacles and create stumbling blocks in your relationships, career, finances, health, and emotions, and in the social spheres of your life. Tracking how Satan seeks to disrupt your Divine path in these areas will allow you to determine the systematic pattern Satan has established to stifle your forward movement in God. As you systematically track your "Satanic obstacles," keep a constant guard when and where temptations or evil manifestations materialize. For instances, you may be particularly vulnerable during certain times of the year because of the anniversary of the death of a loved one, a relationship, or a business. You may be particularly vulnerable during certain stages of your marriage or child-rearing processes. You may be particularly vulnerable when your income/expense ratio hits a certain level. You may be particularly vulnerable when you are dating, or at a specific point during the evolution of a relationship. You may be particularly vulnerable when you are not dating at all. You may be particularly vulnerable when you are under pressure at work.

One thing is certain: you can get sucked into the devil's whirlpool and not know it until it's too late to swim out. In Dante's *Inferno,* hell was described as one concentric circle after another. It's swirling, always swirling, and ever hungry to suck you down to the depths. One theologian described hell as your lifelong accumulation of consequences, resulting from wrong choices. Think about it: one consequence after another, *swirling*. Each and every destructive habit created to cope with consequences adds yet another circle to the swirl. Each habit fed by unresolved, unrecognized issues. *Swirling, always swirling.*

One way to avoid the gravitational pull is to chronicle your temptations. This can reveal to you what Satan already knows about you. And believe me, Satan knows. To effectively combat the devil, you need to know at least as much about yourself as Satan does.

KNOW THYSELF

People who don't know themselves are an open invitation to the devil. You have to truly understand yourself, and I'm not just talking about your good side. I'm talking about knowing your "dark side," that side you'd just as well nobody ever sees, that side of you that you wish you could change, that side that causes you to do things you know are inconsistent with God's Word. Dark sides are those thoughts you think but cannot speak and dare not act on because they will result in your getting fired, disbarred, slapped, embarrassed, fined, jailed, or on the ten o'clock news.

Genealogy, educational training, and income level cannot and do not exempt you or anybody else from having a dark side—or from potentially inflammatory dark side issues! Everyone has a dark side. The ultimate question is this: Do you manage your dark side, or does your dark side manage you? Satan's strategy is to firmly establish your dark side and then encourage you to act out of it, deny it, or be ignorant to its existence. Fall prey to Satan's simple threefold plan and you're in trouble. When Satan knows more about your dark side than you do, then you're cruising for a bruising. Competency minus character equals a potentially Satanic target.

The headlines are a constant barrage of dark-side issues overcoming men and women. When Gary Hart was caught on the bad ship *Monkey Business* with Donna Rice, when Michael Irving was arrested in a motel room with drugs and topless dancers, when Charlie Sheen had his seemingly constant scrapes with the law—these are examples of the dark side at work and play. Public figures are easy targets and popular examples. I hope, however, that you do not allow the transparency of their lives to cause you to overlook your own issues.

The Apostle Paul said, *"The good that I would do, I don't do. That which I don't want to do, I do."* Dark side! This is Satan's playground. This is what he loves to grab hold of! When you don't know what your dark-side issues are, or when you are in denial about them, then you give Satan a target that is entirely too large. The less self-ignorant you are and the more God-conscious you are, the smaller Satan's target is on your backside.

IDENTIFYING YOUR DEMONS

1. How does evil manifest itself in your life?
   - In your social relationships?
   - In your family?
   - In your career?
   - In your self-perception?
2. What are your weaknesses? Your vices?
3. How have your weaknesses caused you to fail yourself and others throughout your life?
4. What weaknesses and vices have you inherited from your family of origin?

THE STRATEGIES OF SATAN

*The foolish never learn from their own mistakes; the wise learn
from the mistakes of others.*

—AFRICAN PROVERB

How do you anticipate Satan's move and timing? The Bible provides a plethora of examples of how Satan moves, showing both his
strategies and motives. Satan is not that smart. He is, however, very
slick. He is not that creative. He is, however, consistent. Most of
Satan's current strategies have their genesis in the Bible. Reading
and understanding Satan's role in the Bible will give you a head
start in safeguarding yourself against him.

Satan blasts through the pages of the Old Testament like some
Terminator in an action movie. John A. Sanford suggests that Satan
makes four official appearances as a supernatural being in the Old
Testament. Let's take a brief look at three of them.

The first appearance is in Zechariah 3:1, in which Satan ap-
pears in his most frequent role—as an accuser. There stands
Joshua, the high priest, with the angel of God on one side and God
Himself watching in defense on the other side. Before them stands
Satan, steadfastly seeking to destroy both Joshua's soul and the an-
gel who acts in Joshua's defense. But standing before God, Satan
has no power to destroy Joshua on his own. He can only *accuse*
Joshua before God, in hopes that God will execute the sentence.

This Biblical example is no faded fantasy; it happens regularly
in our present-day world. Satan will frequently appear before God
in the role of an accuser. He will also hurl accusations through people you may know. Consider this every time someone accuses
you—or you accuse yourself—of being not good enough, smart
enough, tough enough. Could Satan be talking through the accuser? *You bet he could!*

Satan makes his second appearance in I Chronicles 21:1, assuming the role of tempter, encouraging man to break, or go
against, the law of God in order to fulfill a destructive purpose. The
passage retells the story of David, taking a census of the people of
Israel. Because God forbade the counting of heads, this act was
considered a sin. In this Chronicles rendition, Satan stands up
against Israel, provoking David to number its heads. This is yet another ancient story with application in today's world. Satan specializes in encouraging us to disobey God's plan for our lives. While
his strategy will certainly be tantalizing—appealing to the pleasures
of the flesh—Satan's objective is always the same: to kick your
backside! Beware the messengers of temptation! Anything or anybody who encourages you to "go against God" is an instrument of
Satan.

Think of diets you've begun in earnest, only to lose out to the
temptation of sweets. Think of marriages ruined by the temptations of adultery. Think of the money lost because of the temptation of dishonest business dealings. None of us are free from the
devil's infinite tentacles.

Satan makes a third Old Testament appearance in a unique,
history-making, mind-blowing conversation between God and Satan in the first chapter of Job. Satan tells God that Job is faithful
simply because God showers blessings upon him. If God were to
remove the blessings, Satan argues, Job would "turn coat" and forsake God. Satan says Job is in the "God business" for the blessings—money, land, livestock, family—and the blessings only. In
essence, Satan accuses Job of "pimping" God; using God to extract
resources without true loyalty.

Even though God is completely confident of Job's loyalty to
Him, God permits Satan to make an example of Job. In order to
prove Satan wrong, God allows misfortunes to befall Job, and Satan causes Job to suffer immeasurably. But Job was a righteous man

who ultimately kept the Faith, and God replenished his assets seven-fold.

For every Divine action, there seems to be a devilish reaction. God acts; Satan reacts. When our Church, Windsor Village United Methodist Church, gave birth to our AIDS ministry in 1990, a rumor circulated that I had AIDS. (I do not.) When Windsor Village began its Drug Deliverance Ministry in 1989, a rumor circulated that I was both a drug user and a drug pusher. (I have never used or sold drugs.)

All three of these Biblical passages share one common attribute: in each of them, Satan attacks the mind. Maybe you were expecting Satan to stab you with a hot pitchfork, but Satan's style is more insidious and ingenious than that. When he tries to hurt you, he heads for your most vulnerable spot: your mind. Once the evil thoughts are planted there, Satan knows that you can do more harm to yourself than he ever could. With Satan's help, you are definitely your own worst enemy.

And Satan doesn't merely want to make an appearance in your brain. He wants to establish a long-standing stronghold position there. Your mind is his first step to executing a major coup. Give him an inch and he'll attempt to steal a mile. Allow yourself a single, seemingly fleeting evil thought, and like a hungry lion, he'll pounce and sink his jaws into your hide. Worst of all, it's not uncommon for you to not even notice until it's too late.

Think of the businessmen, star athletes, entertainers, preachers, and other public figures who fell from their pinnacles because of lying, deception, manipulation, drugs, alcohol, and adultery. Imagine what sorts of thoughts spun through their minds when they heard the constant praise over their achievement in their respective venues of limelight and public exposure. No doubt they were convinced of their invincibility, which is, of course, an ego-designed gate through which the devil gleefully rides. How could one "little lie" hurt? How could one hit of cocaine possibly hurt? How could one simple tryst with someone else's spouse be a bother? They are, after all, our stars, our Olympians, our best and our brightest.

What happened? In short, they lost touch with themselves. We can imagine their thought patterns: "I'm invincible." "I won't get caught." "My behavior is justified." "I can stop anytime." "This is only temporary." Satan sends the demons of denial to not only knock them off their pedestals, but to kick their backsides. They lost touch with everything that had made them great and had the potential to make them even greater. The philosopher Kierkegaard said, *"The biggest danger, that of losing oneself, can pass off in the world as quietly as if it were nothing; every other loss, an arm, a leg, five dollars, a wife, etc. is bound to be noticed."*

When you're standing atop the mountain of life or when you're down in the valley—that's when you're most vulnerable to Satan. When you're on top of the mountain, Satan can make you think more highly of yourself than you should. When you're down in the valley, Satan can make you think more lowly of yourself than you should. At both extremes, there is the Satanic tendency to create pseudo-gods, false gods, gods of greed, self-pity, anger, addictions, sex, and power. When you find yourself at either point—success or failure—it's particularly urgent to draw near to God.

THE BATTLE IS IN YOUR MIND

The aphorism, "As a man thinketh in his heart, so is he," not only embraces the whole of man's being, but is so comprehensive as to reach out to every condition and circumstance of his life. A man is literally what he thinks, his character being the complete sum of all his thoughts. As the plant springs from, and could not be without, the seed, so every act of a man springs from the hidden seeds of thought . . . man is made or unmade by himself, in the armory of thought he forges the weapons by which he destroys himself; he also fashions tools with which he builds for himself, heavenly mansions of joy and strength and peace. By the right choice and true application of thought, man ascends to the Divine Perfection; by the abuse and wrong application of thought, he descends below the level of beast.

—JAMES ALLEN,
AS A MAN THINKETH

So how can we ward off this Stealth bomber of Evil? First we must learn how to control our thoughts. We've got to assume responsibility for the mental garbage we allow into our brains. When a thought comes into your mind and you know it's no good, when you know it's the work of the devil, don't give it any time. Dismiss it, reject it, and resist it. Martin Luther said, "You cannot keep a bird from flying over your head, but you can keep it from building a nest in your hair." Just because a thought crosses your mind does not mean you have to think about it. You do not have to let just any random thought occupy your mind!

The battle begins in the *mind*. We must make our minds a fortress, a temple so strong that the devil can't find an entrance. The essential question here is "How do you know when a thought is Satanic?" If it does not line up with God's Word, then it is Sa-

tanic. If it doesn't support what God stands for, it's Satanic. What
doesn't glorify God, what doesn't help somebody, what doesn't
take the side of the oppressed, what doesn't support widows and
children and those who have been marginalized by society, is Satanic with a capital S.

Think about Satan's different guises—as accuser, as tempter, as
planter of evil thoughts. When Satan gets into your head, he starts
playing all these roles until you don't know whether you're coming
or going—let alone how to behave, succeed, and glorify the Lord.
First, he'll hit you with those accusations, sending his demons of self-
doubt and his demons of "pass the buck." You all know these
demons: they're the ones who hurl blame—at you and everyone
around you. Then he'll tempt you with ungodly schemes. Finally,
he'll plant evil thoughts in your brain until the growth is so thick it'll
choke the good and productive saplings that are trying to make their
way toward the light. By that time, the holy battle will be all but lost.

THE DEFINITION OF DEMONS

Now, somebody reading this book is asking themselves, *"How can
one Satan destroy so many lives?"* Just as one match can incinerate an
entire forest, Satan burns out lives with sparks that ignite into roaring flames. We've mentioned the concept of demons throughout
this chapter; they're the soldiers in Satan's infinite army of darkness and deceit, serving as both his assistants and his agents. When
Satan was banished from heaven, one-third of the angels in heaven
were banished with him. These are the agents that Satan uses to accomplish his plans for your life. A demon is an evil spirit, and while
technically Christians cannot be "possessed" by evil spirits, evil
spirits can certainly attach themselves to you. Unlike God, the
devil cannot be omnipresent. Arguably, he dispatches e-mails, if
you would, through his agents—demons.

Consider a few examples:

When you make $30,000 a year and spend $35,000, that's a de-mon influencing you. When you're wasting time and money trying to impress other folks with the clothes you're wearing or the car you're driving or the house you're living in, all while your credit cards are overextended and the bill collectors are at your door—that's a demon, or several demons, at work! When you can't go to bed without a drink or a pill, that's a demon stoking the fires of ad-diction! When you're supposed to be in a class, in Church, in syna-gogue, in mosque, in support group, at work, at home, or on a job interview, and you've decided not to show up for some lame excuse, a demon has invaded your decision-making process. When you go to work or Church or out at night dressed as if you're going to a sex session or a pimp's palace or a freak fellowship, that's a demon act-ing as your wardrobe designer. When you and your spouse, or you and your mama and daddy, or you and your sister, brother, or friend start screaming at each other and cannot find an avenue of commu-nication, you've got a demon dancing in your living room. When you and your coworkers are caught in a web of incessant miscom-munication and accusation, then you've got a demon under your desk. When you're making love with your spouse and thinking about somebody else, that's a demon controlling the circuits of your imagination! When you're lying across the couch watching TV at 10:00 P.M. with a bucket of fried chicken in one hand and a washtub of high-fat ice cream in the other—and your doctor has already told you to cut out fat—*Hello!* Twenty-six-year-old grandmothers, thir-teen-year-old crack addicts, fourteen-year-old homicide suspects, forty-year-old soap opera addicts, fifty-year-old layabouts—oh, goodness gracious, the devil and his armies of demons don't care about your name, age, or address. They only want to kick your backside!

Now, when I talk about demons in my sermons, I can see the

signs of denial in dozens of faces. *"I'm not influenced by demons!"* some proclaim.

Let me state this as clearly as I can: If you are alive and breathing, evil spirits are going to mess with you.

Demons, I've discovered, come in many varieties:

PERSONAL DEMONS

Vanity, greed, sloth, adultery, envy, despair—all are the fallen fruit on which personal demons feed. It was, of course, vanity that incited the devil to rebel against God in the first place. In Milton's *Paradise Lost*, as Lucifer and his fallen legion of demons establish their underworld kingdom after the Almighty expelled them from heaven, we hear the Prince of Darkness announce:

> *"Here we may reign secure, and in my choice*
> *To reign is worth ambition though in hell:*
> *Better to reign in hell than serve in heaven."*

When we surrender to vanity, or to its related personal demons, we are, like the legendary Faust, signing a contract with the devil. When our blind desire for money obstructs our responsibilities as spouses and parents, we have signed our names along the dotted line of the devil's contract. When we point to historical ledgers of racial oppression or gender bias as grounds for mediocrity, we have taken the pen from Satan and scribbled our name on his contract. When we practice or endorse prejudice based upon ethnocentrism, we are signing up with the devil. When we think we're so sexy, cool, hip, or hot that we see "no problem" in acting out our lustful desires to sleep with our neighbor's spouse or "borrow" our boss's money, we have agreed to enlist our services with the devil. When we gnash our teeth with envy as our colleagues, associates, and acquaintances pass us on the ladder of success, the devil rubs his hands together in delight, knowing he has persuaded us to sign our names to that vile contract.

SOCIAL DEMONS

When confronting the devil, we must also address what the author Walter Wink calls "social demons." Personal demons attack individuals. Social demons permeate our social and economic structures. Here I'm talking about racism, classism, ageism, ethnocentrism, materialism, and sexism. Social demons work not only in the mean streets, but also in the hallways of so-called "respectability." You don't need 20/20 vision to see their victims on the corner, selling drugs, or in the crack houses, or in the hallways of the homeless shelters, where they have planted deadly seeds of decay and despair. Social demons are sneaky. They'll pop into your day like jack-in-the-boxes in places you'd never suspect. They lurk in the loan departments of banks, where there are a hundred nos for every yes. They haunt the offices of mortgage firms. They prowl the corridors of government and corporate America. And as they hide under the auspices of "respectability," they watch and listen, all set to pounce on their next victim.

We've got social demons at our local elementary school. I am told that, at a recent faculty meeting, one teacher stood up and said, "We want to continue to have separate PTAs here for the vanguard students and another for the regular kids. We want to continue to have separate schools within this one school, because if we combine the vanguard program with the regular program, if we allow all the children to attend PE or eat lunch together or sit with one another in the same classrooms, then the intelligence level of the entire school will drop."

DECOY DEMONS

Labeled by my wife, Suzette, these decoy demons are demons of distraction that are so creative in dropping seemingly delicious options in our path. Decoy demons hide in the hallways and whisper your name from the shadows. They want to compel you into taking some seemingly minor diversion that will throw you off your path anywhere from a few hours to a lifetime. Decoy demons are experts at showing you shortcuts that go nowhere, easier routes to the top that take you straight to the bottom. Decoy demons entice you to major in the minor and minor in the major. They specialize in distracting and derailing. As Charles Stith, U.S. Ambassador to Tanzania, says, "You must keep the main thing the main thing." Decoy demons specialize in sidetracking you from your God-given vision and mission.

DEMONS OF DISOBEDIENCE

When you are disobedient, Satan gets the glory, and he has ways of making disobedience look good! He'll cook you like you cook a frog. You don't put a frog in hot water; he'll hop right out. You put a frog in cool water, then turn up the heat . . . *slowly.* That's the way the devil cooks us with his demons of disobedience. He puts us in a pot of seeming pleasure, then begins to turn up the heat. He makes disobedience look sweet, delicious, delightful, and just like the water, *cool.* He'll appeal to your eyes, taste buds, and carnal pleasures. Then, just when it's too late to hop out of his pot, you're cooked and ready for him to devour.

DEFEATING YOUR DEMONS

1. Let go of your negative attitudes, friendships, and self-defeating behaviors. For every identifiable demon, stage a Comeback (Chapter 2) to overcome it.
2. Make a list of the demons, however minute, that you feel have some control over your life. Post that list in a place where you can see it daily, then take concentrated effort to rid your life of demonic influences in these areas.
3. Take time to discuss your weakness and vices with the "Nathans" in your life. Remember, evil loves darkness; throw open the light on your life. Let others know what's going on inside. You have supporters around you. But you may not find them if you don't ask.

DEFEATING YOUR DEMONS

Put on the whole armor of God, that ye shall be able to stand against the wiles of the Devil.

—EPHESIANS 6:11

Okay, now that we know what Satan is, and how he can attack us, let's get down to whuppin' him. The devil *is* eminently *"whupable."* You read me right: he's whupable! There's even a road map to whuppin' him, a battle plan that spells out exactly how to drive the devil away from your life. To find it, turn to Ephesians 6:10–20, which outlines humankind's fight to the finish with the devil and identifies the armaments that we can call upon to help ensure victory.

In this instructive Bible passage, Paul describes a full military vestment—*a veritable full metal jacket against the devil!*—that, properly assembled and worn, allows humankind, then and now, to defeat the wicked wiles of the devil and thwart his agenda.

The armor described in Ephesians 6:10–20 is actually comparable to the armor God Himself wears. In Isaiah 59:17, the implication is clear. If God symbolically wears armor when opposing a power, then we'd better suit up as well. Every part of the body that's vulnerable to the enemy should be covered. Here is the armor, taken verbatim from Ephesians, the warrior's impenetrable vestment, that can become your ultimate protection against the devil. I realize that this isn't strictly a literal interpretation of the Biblical text, but I hope it will be useful nonetheless.

Stand with truth as a belt around your waist. The ancient soldiers wore a sword on their belts, which gave them strength against their enemies. The belt was a sign that they were prepared for battle. In your fight against evil in the modern world, preparedness is a critical condition for victory. The first step in becoming prepared is to see and know the truth about yourself and your situation. Be assured that Satan is prepared for battle. If you're deluding yourself in any of the myriad ways in which many of us find it so easy to delude ourselves, then the battle is over before it begins. In other words, look through the veil of denial and see yourself as you truly are.

Wear the breastplate of Righteousness. In the Bible, the warrior's breastplate, made of metal, protected the chest and the throat. From a Christian perspective, Righteousness was found in and through Jesus. In fact, Jesus was viewed *as* Righteousness. In your modern-day war against evil, Righteousness is the breastplate that protects your heart. Individuals with a righteous heart are not only impenetrable to the wiles of the devil; they are positioning themselves to live a blessed life as well. When you are righteous, you are living a life beyond doubt, and the devil cannot destroy you.

Righteousness is the active interpretation of Faith. Living anything other than a righteous life is evidence that the devil is well into his work.

The breastplate of Righteousness reminds us of God's call to social redress. It is morally incongruent, if not hypocritical, to claim to love your neighbor without being committed to justice and fairness in society. The same devil who seeks to sow havoc within you also seeks to sow havoc among us. Check yourself. Do you automatically or intrinsically dislike, distrust, or even abhor an individual simply because of his or her ethnicity or social background? As long as you harbor demons of ethnocentrism, the devil will make certain that your productivity is beneath your God-given potential.

Wear the shoes of peace. The ancient soldier wore sandals, which signified that he was suited up and ready for battle. In today's world, the shoes of peace similarly signify that we are suited up and ready to march to become the best that we can be. Pay special attention to this: In order for your armor to accomplish the purpose for which it was designed, you must mobilize for action. Don't suit up in your armor for appearance purposes; always be ready to move! The shoes represent your readiness for the journey from where you are to where God wants you to be. The shoes are the bedrock. Even while God provides us with stronger armor—a helmet, a breastplate, and a shield—without shoes we couldn't move. God clearly expects us to be willing, participatory workers, not sideline observers. God is calling you to be a participant, not a spectator.

In all things, take Faith as a shield, for with it you will be able to quench the flaming darts of the evil one. Now we're getting into the heavy armor: the shield of Faith. This is Paul's most potent protection. The ancient warriors carried a large quadrangular shield made of wood and frequently drenched in water to guard against and extinguish the enemy's fiery darts. In our war against evil, we must also wear Faith as a shield against the fiery darts of the devil. Faith—which I recently heard described as Fantastic Adventures in Trusting Him—can become an impenetrable shield against whatever the devil hurls our way.

Put on the helmet of Salvation. One of our most powerful weapons is not exterior armor but the decision to obey and trust God. The "helmet of Salvation" referred to in Ephesians is, of course, Salvation through Christ. But no matter your denomination or Faith, it's critical to realize that Satan's first target is the mind. Therefore, wear the helmet which protects the decision point of your belief system: your mind. Safeguard your mind from the continuous bombarding of potentially evil temptations that you will encounter daily. Put your helmet on!

Take the Sword of the Spirit, which is the Word of God. Up until this point, the armor of God has been defensive: truth as a belt; Righteousness as a breastplate; peace as shoes; Faith as a shield; Salvation as a helmet. But now we are given an *offensive* weapon against evil. The Sword of the Spirit—the Word of God—to be wielded against the devil. As it says in Hebrews 4:12: "The Word of God is living and active; sharper than any two-edged sword, dividing soul and spirit, joints and marrow." Become a never-ending student of God's Word; it can and will show you the way. The Bible, in 2 Timothy 3:16–17, informs us that "all scripture is given by inspiration of God, and is profitable for doctrine, for reproof, for correction, for instruction, for righteousness, that the man of God may be complete, thoroughly equipped for every good work."

Finally, it is written in Ephesians to "keep praying in the spirit on all occasions, with all kind of prayers and entreaties to God." Prayer is not necessarily part of the armor of God; but prayer sanctifies every aspect of the armor. Without prayer, the armor is rendered impotent. With this in mind, be alert and always keep on praying for all the saints. For Paul, prayer is the greatest ongoing weapon against the devil. In Ephesians, he details three ways to release the power of prayer:

1. Prayer must be constant, daily, not reserved for times of crisis.
2. Prayer must be intense, bold, done with complete concentration and confidence.
3. Prayer must be unselfish, uniting humankind with the community.

The last point is particularly important. We have to learn to fight the devil in our community, and family. If you've read the Old Testament, you know that the Israelites, and even the God of the Old Testament, did not separate love for an individual from justice in society. For them, it was impossible to harbor love for an individual without the application of justice, just as it was impossible to apply justice in society without love for the individual. The two have gone together since time immemorial.

VICTORY OVER SATAN

There are two types of people in this world: those who get up and the demons run to them and those who get up and the demons run away from them. It's not rocket science to know which person attracts what.

I can hear the demons now: *"Ooh, she's up again! I'm gonna whup her behind today! She thought she caught a whuppin' yesterday, but her 'worst' is yet to come!"*

Wherever there is reigning doubt, denial, low self-esteem, envy—in short, whenever and wherever there is an absence or mistrust of God—Satan, most assuredly, is not only residing but presiding. As our world grows smaller and smaller and evil continues to rear its ugly head from the shadows of our city streets and suburban neighborhoods, we need to understand and learn to overcome the devil and his cumbersome webs of illusion and accusation. And believe me, as soon as you separate yourself from the pack, the devil will try to drag you down.

Your soul can be saved, but if you are not perpetually on guard, the devil will know where to strike you and then keep on striking you. If Satan knows you have a warped work ethic, he will help you work yourself to death. If Satan knows you are looking at life through the dirty lenses of doubt and negativity, he will show you an ugly world. If Satan knows that material possessions give you a thrill, he'll exile you to a life of shopping malls and credit or debit cards, until you're literally buried under the weight of the things you thought you loved. If Satan knows that fattening foods or alcohol are your weakness, he will lay out a feast before you that will wreck your health and destroy your sobriety. If Satan knows you are an "attention addict," he will consistently attempt to persuade you that you are underappreciated by those whose opinions you value. If Satan knows that you are wrestling with low self-esteem, then he will tempt you to compare yourself with others.

The devil knows where you live. He'll seize you in schools, shopping malls, bars, offices, even in the privacy of your own home. Let the devil get that first grip, and it will turn into a stranglehold. Pick up the devil as a hitchhiker and he'll soon want to drive. Pretty soon, you'll be gnashing your teeth, turning rigid, inflexible, cantankerous, negative, racist . . . Before you realize it, you'll be too old and ornery to pull out of the tailspin. You'll be grateful for death.

Death will seem like recess after a few study sessions with the devil. It happens every day in every city in countless lives.

I preside over far too many funerals. I sometimes ask the director, "How many young folk funerals are you doing nowadays?"

"Ah, pastor," comes the heavyhearted reply, "an unprecedented number!"

When I ask what these youths are dying from, the answers are a litany of Satanic influences: homicide, heart attack, alcohol, drugs . . . the list is, I am frequently told, "very long and very tragic, pastor."

The devil doesn't sort by age. He is an equal-opportunity destroyer. Once he separates parents from their children, he turns his hungry eyes to youth, because he knows full well how vulnerable they are with little or no guidance at home. The devil knows that if he can wipe out the youth of today, he won't have to worry about the adults of tomorrow. If youth is left to his devices, there won't be any adults of tomorrow! If we continue to neglect giving our children the wisdom and guidance they need to conquer the devil, our sons and daughters may never see the sun of a new day.

KILLING SOME GIANTS

"Behold, I have given you power to tread on snakes and scorpions, and upon every power of the enemy—nothing will harm you!"
—LUKE 10:18–19

After you've begun to whup the devil, you're going to have to kill some Giants.

Now, somebody reading this book is asking, "What's the difference between the devil and a Giant?" The devil is a spirit, the prince of evil. A Giant is anything or anybody which or who is preventing you from pursuing or receiving what God wants you to have or being who God wants you to be.

A Giant could be considered an offspring, offshoot, or evil offering of the devil. If the devil influences the thoughts, habits, and temptations that steer us wrong or hold us back—shame, embarrassment, self-destruction—Giants are all the tangible "things" that we fail to overcome because we *think* we can't. Giants are seemingly unattainable goals, the unfinished objectives, the unfulfilled dreams that keep us mired in the mediocre when God meant for us to rise to the top.

Any great undertaking begins with a steady slaying of giants, ranging from David vs. Goliath to Holyfield vs. Tyson to an ordinary American trying to get his G.E.D. A Giant is anything or anybody that keeps you from being who God intended you to be or doing what God intended you to do. A Giant may be the size of a gnat or the head of a pin. But if your Faith is smaller than that gnat or that head of a pin, then your Giant is going to be insurmountable in your mind. The Giant may be inside of you or outside, tangible or intangible, physical or emotional, educational or career-oriented. The Giant could be a habit, attitude, belief, family-origin issue, philosophy, perception, or person that or who stands between you and God, between who you are and who God wants you to be, between where you are and where God wants you to be, between what you believe and what God wants you to believe.

In the case of our Church, the Giant was the incongruent image that we had to constantly fight and overcome: that Churches are solely centers of prayer, not economic development. You, too, have to battle misconceptions—imposed by yourself and by others—that will strive to categorize, belittle, or limit you! Anything that tries to make you smaller than you can be is a Giant. And like the devil, Giants are whupable. How? By following the examples of other Giant killers. Let's discuss a few of the steps inspired by the teachings of John Maxell, former pastor at Skyline Weslyan Church in San Diego, now a Church consultant headquartered in Atlanta, Ga.

Giant killers learn how to see victory in the bowels of defeat. Every fight is a test: can you turn a positive into a negative? We are all engaged in some kind of fight, either coming out of or going into one, on a constant basis. You don't have to look too far to see the effect on those who have given up fighting. Whenever you see folks whose lives are a constant pity party, those with a consistent complaint coming out of their mouths, those for whom nothing is ever going right, they've given up the fight. But a life without battle is little life at all. Where there's no conflict, there's no growth. I've discovered that there are three components to every fight: you, your opponent (whether it's a person, a system, or a thing), and God. If you can rely on God as your constant ally, you will begin to see your Giants as nothing but tools that God may use to fashion, develop, nurture, and grow you.

One way to befuddle and confuse those who will try to limit you is to keep your integrity and enthusiasm even when the walls seem to be crumbling around you. A Giant can introduce you to the deeper levels of yourself. When you're battling something bigger than you are, you may discover that you yourself are bigger than you realized. Look at it this way, Giant annihilation is actually an exercise in self-esteem. The more Giants you defeat, the more confident you're going to feel when another one comes along.

Giant killers don't start out as Giant killers. If you're a little unprepared about assuming the role of Giant killer, realize that nobody is totally prepared to slay giants in the beginning. In the Bible, David didn't wake up one morning and immediately kill Goliath. If you'll read 1 Samuel 16, you'll see that David was a meek musician. If you'll turn to 1 Samuel 17, you'll see where David began to take care of the sheep. But David was ever faithful over the small things: taking care of his musical instrument, watching over his sheep. There is a supreme lesson in this: Become a master over the small things. Do you think Michael Jordan started out shooting three-pointers the moment he leaped from his mother's womb? No. He started out with the small things. He got cut from his high school basketball team. He didn't start out as a giant killer. But he didn't give up the fight. Cherish the small things. Master them. They will grow large.

Giant killers know that the reward is always greater than the risk. Repeat after me: The potential is always greater than the problem, the objective is always bigger than the objection, God is always more powerful than the giant. I'm not talking about being deaf, dumb, or blind to your reality. I'm merely talking about being "God-conscious" enough to know that whatever giant you're fighting, the reward is always going to be greater than the risk. Satan specializes in blinding us to the rewards; he magnifies the risks ten-fold, causing us to sit on our Humpty-Dumpty behinds *and do nothing.* If you have been waiting for all your fear to leave prior to attacking your giants, reconsider your situation based on this reality: Faith is not the absence of fear. Faith propels you forward in spite of fear. Fear is a weapon that Satan uses to paralyze you. Remember, Satan's arsenal is no match for God's. Trust God to help you. Follow God's leadership. Depend upon God for your deliverance, and CHARGE that giant!

Giant killers realize that Giants are representatives of deeper issues. Folks had more sense about fighting wars in the days when David fought Goliath. They said, "There's no need in countless men losing their lives, so let's choose one representative from each nation to step forward and engage in war." Victory would go to whichever individual won the battle for their nation as a whole. That's why for forty days and forty nights, Goliath stepped forward and asked, "Who will challenge me today?" Just like Goliath was representing an entire community, the Giants in your life never stand alone. They represent other issues, deeper issues. If your Giant is overeating, there are certainly other issues driving your overeating. If your Giant is smoking, there are other psychological issues driving your smoking. Whether it's fear, alcoholism, emotional detachment, there are deeper, darker issues associated with that Giant. Realize that behind each Giant lie its causes: pain, guilt, shame. Fight the underlying causes and you will topple the Giant.

One word of warning: watch out for the critics. They're going to surround your life like cackling birds, crowing negatives. Always remember that you are on a mission from God, and God has not called you to live up to the expectations of some zip-up-the-back, round-the-corner, moose-breath, pigeon-toed cookie who is not, will not, and probably never will have the guts to step up and fight their own Giants. To these folks, you must make an announcement: *This train is leaving the station. You have three options: work with me and ride on the train; get your excess-baggage self off the train; or finally, get in front of the train and I'll roll right over you. But this train is leaving the station . . . NOW!* You have things to do, missions to accomplish, places to go. You don't have time to suck up to Satan's folks. Just as you can't expect blood to come out of a turnip or an orange tree to produce grapes or a cow to give birth to a squirrel, you can't expect small-minded, Satanic, evil-spirited folks to say good things about you when you're out there slaying Giants. So forget that expectation—and move on!

Giant killers are not overwhelmed by the challenge. Satan destroys many of us through intimidation. I'm reminded of the legendary baseball pitching great Walter Johnson, who had an earned-run average of less than 2. During one game, when Johnson faced a trembling rookie, he threw a sizzling curve ball that cut across the plate like a fireball. *Strike one!* The second pitch was even more miraculous, a looping end shoot that broke in off the outside corner. *Strike two!* The rookie, eyes swirling, took the bat off his shoulder and slumped off toward the dugout. "Wait a minute!" said the umpire. "You have three strikes before you're out. You've only had two!" The rookie shook his head. "Naw," he spat. "Standing there for the third pitch isn't going to do me any good. I can't see the ball. I can't hit the ball. I'm going back to the dugout." Somebody reading this book is in the same position as that rookie. You're overwhelmed by the army of Giants that life has placed in your path. You've aborted your Giant-killing processes and retreated to the dugout. How do you get out? You examine the pitches one at a time and keep swinging, focusing on each pitch, never allowing your past failures to shackle the expectations of the present.

Giant killers build on past successes. In the Bible, David said, "When I was taking care of the sheep, a lion came up and I whipped his behind. Then, a bear came up and I whipped the bear. And the same God that blessed me to beat the bear is the same God who blessed me to whip the lion is the same God who is going to bless me to beat Goliath." There is power in past successes. This power, if wielded correctly, can become a tangible fuel to enable you to move on to greater victories. Remember, earlier in this book, when I talked about the speech impediment that plagued me through elementary and part of junior high school? How did I get over it? *I spoke.* That's how you whup a Giant! If it's a speech impediment, you speak. If it's a work impediment, you work! If it's a Faith impediment, you pray! If it's a strength impediment, you exercise! Do the thing that's trying to whup you and you will become master over it. Remember: *An individual who has the right mix of God-confidence and self-confidence is indestructible.* They can convert enemies into stepping stones, evil into good, Giants into accomplishments.

Giant killers create their own style. When David prepared to fight

Goliath, Saul dressed him in Saul's uniform. David tried it on and it did not fit. Nothing fit. Finally, David said, "Wait a minute! This isn't going to work! This is your stuff, Saul. But you're not going into battle. I am! I've got to wear my own clothes." Of course, Saul would have gone up against Goliath with a *real* weapon—maybe even an arsenal of weapons. David, in his singular style, didn't need a shield or a javelin. He only needed only five stones, a slingshot, and the God-confidence that he could get the job done. Somebody reading this book is sitting on her God-given Giant-killing capabilities because she's waiting for the Lord to bless them in the way she's seen Him bless somebody else. But God has already given you everything you need to go forth in battle. Just like David, you have your own weapons and armor, your own style. Like David, draw a line in the sand and stand up to the evil that is denying you the life you deserve. God anointed David to defeat Goliath with the slingshot. Had young David used Saul's clothes or weapons, David's life would have been in real danger.

Now, somebody reading this book is thinking, "If David has so much Faith, why did he need five stones?" That's a good question. The answer is that Goliath had four brothers! Not only is God willing and able to defeat our enemies, He'll even prepare you for future battles that may never occur.

One of the greatest demons you will probably ever fight is one you come in contact with every single day. It may even have more temptation swirling around it than any other area of your life. But once conquered, this demon can become the source of enormous joy. Until then, you'll have to use all your devil-whuppin' techniques to slay it. But it's a foe that's absolutely whupable.

I'm talking, of course, about the demonic love of *money*.

To take the first step toward financial fulfillment, curse the demons of doubt and turn the page.

5

❧

Creating Wealth God's Way

*Wealth is not in making money, but in making the (wo)man
while (s)he is making money.*

—JOHN WICKER

*"But seek first His kingdom and His righteousness, and all these
things will be given to you as well."*

—MATTHEW 6:33

TO SUMMON FORTH SOME DEMONS, ALL YOU HAVE TO DO IS say one word aloud: *Money!* It's like flashing a bankroll on a busy big-city street corner. The devil swirls around the matter of money like a giant bat in a small, dark cave. We're going to throw some light on that cave now. We're going to blast through its thick stone walls and open it up to the light. As it says in the Book of Psalms, unless there is economic justice, there will be no peace in the community. Unless there is peace in the community, there will be no peace among the individuals. If there's no peace among the individuals, then Satan has one more welcome mat to walk across. Without economic power—or the promise of economic power—there is no hope.

In this chapter, we're going to learn God's mathematics, a simple, yet practical formula for creating, and keeping, financial abundance in your life.

Remember in Chapter 2, when I told you about growing up in the Fifth Ward of Houston, and watching the "materially blessed" folks on the fringes of the law having a disproportionate amount of prosperity? I said that through the mindset of a high school student, who was admittedly influenced by material goods, the so-called "bad folks" seemed to be overblessed. There I was, watching the pimps, prostitutes, hustlers, and pigeon droppers driving new cars and wearing diamonds and fashionable clothes, while so many of the so-called "spiritual folks" appeared to be struggling. There was a gap in my mind between being "religious" and "being prosperous," which was underlined by some churchgoing folk who subscribed to the notion that you had to be broke in order to be holy.

Since that time, two salient realizations have occurred to me, which have had a tremendous impact on my evolution. First, having a relationship with God is infinitely more important than being "religious." This is an important distinction to make. Religious folk are connected with institutions; relationship folk are connected to God. Religious folk tend to hold on to the status quo; relationship folk are open to God doing a "new thing" in them (à la Isaiah). Religious folk are predisposed to pleasing Church people; relationship folk are predisposed to pleasing God through their own actions. As you will discover in this chapter, these distinctions are crucial. Additionally, the characteristics of "relationship folk" are a necessary condition in taking your financial life to the next level in God.

Secondly, I realized I was born to be blessed. I realized that God wants to bless me! He has chosen me for His blessings. Wow! That was one incredible realization. I really believe—and thus am able to receive—these declarations. Whether I deserve the blessings is beside the point: Blessings are based on God's grace, not on merit. Grace, by definition, cannot be earned. While we certainly want to avoid what the nineteenth-century German theologian Dietrich Bonhoeffer called "Cheap Grace," which can be defined as basically taking God's grace for granted, God's economy of blessings is not based upon meritocracy. I'm blessed! And God wants to bless you, too.

Sparking these two important realizations was that Biblical passage we've discussed from Joshua 1:8: *"The book of law shall not depart from your mouth, but you shall meditate in it day and night, that you may observe to do according to all that is written in it, for then you will make your way prosperous. And you will have good success."*

When I began to focus on God's perspective on money, I realized it was different from society's view of God's perspective on money. For instance, more than half of the parables told by Jesus in the New Testament deal with money. The Bible states that "the love of money is the root of evil," not money in itself. In fact, in some communities, as Dr. Floyd Flake, the pastor of Allen Temple A.M.E. Church in Queens, New York, states, "It's the *lack* of money that is the root of evil." When you combine the lack of money with the greed of money, it's easy to understand why negative emotions run rampant when the M word is mentioned!

HOW THE BLESSINGS COULD BECOME A CURSE

If you want to understand how the love of money or the lack of money can become the root of all evil, you must first understand the concept of blessings. In many ways, blessings were, and still are, the original currency. God initially intended the medium of exchange—gold, silver, and eventually, money—to be used as a blessing. Almost immediately, however, human beings allowed Satan to warp their perspective, thus turning what God intended to be a blessing into a curse. Whenever you use money for the wrong reasons, its blessings are tainted, wasted, or worse.

The love of money for its own sake flows away from God, not

toward God. We have exalted money to mean far more than God initially intended, which, in part, is why demons latch on to it so effectively. Some of us make money a "pseudo-God," the worship of which always leads to trouble. Whenever humans remove a blessing from its intended purpose, rest assured the devil will exacerbate the situation by maximizing its potential for evil.

We all know how the pursuit of money often brings out the *absolute* worst in some people. But avoiding the subject is a sure route to colliding head-first with financial trouble. We must not allow our institutionalized "dark-side" perspective of money to be cast upon God. God has plenty of guidance to shine upon the subject. It's our duty to learn it and heed His words. When we view money through the lens of God, we will grow in God's blessedness and be a blessing to those we appreciate.

When I read Joshua 1:8 and began to reflect on the matter of God and money, I knew, then and there, that God wanted his followers to be prosperous and have good success. God did not make provisions—whether it's stocks and bonds, nice cars and nice homes, or peace of mind, joy, and healthy self-esteem—for Satan's kids! These provisions are for His children, if they are for anybody!

It sounded so right on paper. But then, in June 1993, my congregation and I met the Satan of silver right in our own backyard. We'd been seriously blessed, deeded with 25 acres of land by Fiesta, Inc., to build our Power Center. But just as every privilege comes with a responsibility, the deed came with a provision. We had to raise the money to renovate the vacant 104,000-square-foot old Kmart building and operate what would become a $10 million blessing to the community, The Power Center. Fiesta, Inc.'s gracious donation, spearheaded by Fiesta's chairman, Donald Bonham, was the first of its kind in the State of Texas. Triggered by Windsor Village's reputation for community service, Fiesta's contribution is an excellent example of how private enterprise can balance the corporate push for profits with a real and lasting compassion for people. Fiesta's contribution was valued at $4.2 million. Thank God for Mr. Bonham and Fiesta!

Nonetheless, as it's written in the Bible, "unto whom much is given, much is expected." Fiesta's history-making contribution set the stage for how private enterprises and nonprofit entities can collaborate to make an indelibly Divine difference in the community. Giving birth to The Power Center was an epic struggle, a sterling example of how God helps those who help themselves. When the architects told us the price—$2.6 million—we were momentarily staggered. The cost would end up being considerably more than that, but the figure was plenty to start with. We were a volunteer board of five people, none of whom, as individuals, had any experience in raising $2.6 million for a community project! We consisted of an attorney (Genora Boykins), a human resources manager (Al Scarborough), a housewife (Maude Collins), an accountant (J. Otis Mitchell), and me.

The devil would try to shroud us in a cloud of doubt. After all, that's his job. We would have to face him down before we could move on. Our doubts would literally hold us captive. We had to plunge forward into a world where few congregations had ever gone before.

But we had one thing in our corner, just as you do in your own personal crusade. The Bible has more to say about money than Peter Lynch, the Motley Fool, and a passel of stock prognosticators combined. Upon intelligent reflection, Jesus frequently used money to describe the meaning, characteristics, and dynamics of the Kingdom of God. You might call it God's Mathematics for financial abundance. The equation goes something like this:

$$\text{Faith} + \text{Good Stewardship} + \text{Giving} = \text{Abundance.}$$

Let's examine the three points in sequence.

FAITH

That the trial of your faith, being more precious than of gold that
perishes, though it be tried with fire . . .
                                        —1 PETER 1:7

What if I told you that you're already wealthy, that you don't have
to want for anything, that there's an abundant bank account with
your name on it awaiting you and all you have to do to access it is to
believe that it exists?

"*What's the catch?*" you might immediately ask.

But there's no catch, no fine print, no duplicitous clauses.

Here, in short, is "the deal": The world and all its abundance
belong to God. What we give back to Him—Faith, prayer, and personal sacrifice—is the "rent" we pay for using God's resources.
What we receive and how we receive depends on how much we are
prepared to give. In this way, you've already been blessed abun-
dantly, although perhaps not in the way you imagine. You've been
blessed to be a blessing to yourself and others. When God blessed
you, He did not have you specifically in mind. Almighty God expects His blessings to flow *through* you to those around you. The
more blessings that flow through you, the more He bestows. Depending on how you are to me, so I will be to you, God reveals in
Jeremiah.

Many people never receive God's blessings, because they have
a warped perspective of either God or themselves or both. They
never realize God is the Supply and the Supplier of their resources.
So when they don't receive His blessings, they fall prey to low self-
esteem and feelings of unworthiness. They stay stalled in lower
economic strata, in dead-end jobs and self-destructive spending
habits.

Others fall victim to allowing Satan to define them according to
how much they earn or how much they're worth financially. Grow-

ing up in a culture that thrives on capitalism, the work ethic, and the "America's Business Is Business" principle, it is easy to slip into one of the devil's traps: your self-esteem becomes salary-esteem. In other words, how you perceive yourself and what you think about yourself is a function of how much money you earn. Don't misunderstand: I fully endorse accountability and responsibility, but it is unhealthy to entangle your sense of worth in the web of dollars.

Your worth, as a member of God's creation, is not dependent on the workplace's assessment of your economic "value added-ness," and how much someone is willing to pay to secure your services or the right to access your knowledge. If you allow your self-esteem to ride on the roller coaster of employment or unemployment, fat bonuses or lean bonuses, entrepreneurial reward or corporate bust, then you are positioning yourself for disappointment, disgust, and depression. If you allow your self-esteem to ride this roller coaster, you also position yourself for self-aggrandizement, false pride, and an inflated ego. Satan, the master counterfeiter, can pummel you into the bowels of disappointment when you are broke. Or he can rocket you into the atmosphere of arrogance when the money is flowing. Temptation should be resisted at both altitudes. Your self-worth is a function of who you are in God, not what you own!

If you recognize any of these characteristics in yourself, practice the first principle of God's Mathematics: Faith.

If the essence of prayer is communicating with God and receiving God's primary will for your life, then Faith is the belief that God is going to answer those prayers. It's an inner knowing that it's going to be done. Faith provides the motivation and focus to survive when all else fails. I don't care if you're broke as the Ten Commandments, even when you have absolutely nothing in the way of material possessions, you still have the ability to *believe*. No one can deny you your power to believe!

But as we've discussed, hand in hand with Faith comes action.

Allow me to tell you two very different stories that illustrate the power of Faith, especially in regard to our search for God's abundance.

The first story is about a woman who had gone shopping at a grocery store near the Astrodome, in Houston. Walking into the store, she noticed a woman sitting in a car, slumped over the steering wheel. When my friend had finished her shopping, she returned to find the woman still slumped over the steering wheel. She could see into the back seat, where there was a sack of groceries, atop which, she noticed, was a broken-open can of biscuits.

My friend walked up the woman slumped over her steering wheel.

"Lady, are you all right?" she asked.

"Can't you see that blood on my back?" the woman replied. *"Call an ambulance!"*

My friend looked at the woman's back, then told her that she didn't see any blood.

But the woman was insistent. "I've been shot!" she exclaimed.

My friend pointed to the broken-open tin of biscuits in the back seat.

"Lady, you haven't been shot!" she said. "You've been hit by a biscuit!"

A can of biscuits had exploded and one of the biscuits had flown from the can and hit the lady at the bottom of her neck. The basic story serves to illustrate a deeper, instructive truth. As I began to reflect on the story, I came to the conclusion that so many of us are just like that lady slumped over her steering wheel. God has granted us the power and the authority to take our key of trust and insert it into the ignition of Faith, to turn that key and begin the glorious journey of God's primary will for our lives. But instead of driving in the direction of our God-given Vision, a lot of us are stuck in the driver's seat, with the engine turned off, slumped over the steering wheel, pulverized, mesmerized, and otherwise stalled. Thinking we've been shot by a bullet when we've only been hit by biscuit!

You see, *fear* had overcome that woman. When the can exploded, it sounded like a gun—*to her.* When the biscuit hit her on the back of the neck, it felt like a bullet—*to her.* So she figured, *"If it sounds like a gun and feels like a bullet, I must've been shot! So I'll just sit here and wait for my change to come."*

I recently read an interesting listing of the "Seven Levels of Fear" by Mike Donahue of Colorado Mountain School. Here are the seven levels he identified, in descending order: Paralysis (fear of doing the wrong things), Inefficiency (fear of doing the right things wrong), Catastrophizing (fear of things getting worse), Holding On (fear of letting go), Self-doubt (fear of not being physically able), Normalcy (fear of being different), and Disbelief (fear of the unknown). To combat these fears, Donahue suggests instituting what he calls "The Seven Levels of Change." Here are the seven levels he identifies: Effectiveness (doing the right things), Efficiency (doing things right), Improving (doing things better), Cutting (doing away with things you don't need), Copying (doing things others are doing), Being Different (doing things no one else is doing), and Breakout! (doing things that can't be done). Notice that all seven levels of fear are passive, without action. But each of the levels of change begins with the word "doing." Here's a subtle yet important thing to note: Fear is fed by inaction; change always begins with action.

As I've indicated before, FEAR is the acronym for False Evidence Appearing Real. You may be spiritually, relationally, emotionally, psychologically, socially and most of all, financially slumped over your steering wheel, pulverized by fear. But let me assure you of this: You have not been shot by a bullet, you've just been hit by a biscuit. You've just been fired from your job, and Satan wants you to lose your mind.

You feel as if you've been struck by a bullet. But no! You've just been hit by a biscuit. You just had your boyfriend or girlfriend walk out on you, and your whole world revolved around him or her.

You think you've been struck by a bullet. No, no, no. You've just been hit by a biscuit.

Satan is proficient at making reality look like fantasy and making fantasy look like reality. He can take the truth and make it look like a lie, and a lie like the truth. He can make your assets look like liabilities and your liabilities look like assets. He makes your strengths look like weaknesses and your weaknesses look like strengths. My prayer for you, before we go any further, is this: The Lord will always bless you to know the difference between bullets and biscuits. Trusting God is the first step. But there's more: The devil wants you slumped over that steering wheel, thinking you've got blood on our back, just waiting around to die. But you have to realize the devil's only throwing biscuits; the only bullets he can fire are those you create for him in your own mind.

Now, I'm not saying there aren't real bullets in life. Let's assume you've been victimized by the worst economic situation imaginable. And we're talking bullets, not biscuits. The truth of the matter is that if you still have the presence of mind to be reading this chapter, then there is hope! Do not allow Satan to destroy your expectation for a better tomorrow based on your disappointments of today. Let's access the appropriate resources so that the bullet that has temporarily maimed you can be removed, your wounds can be bandaged, and your life can be resumed, new and improved!

As the Bible reminds us in Hebrews 11, "now faith is the substance of things hoped for, the evidence of things not seen." It is absolutely crucial to check what you're hoping for. It's important to hope for things that are consistent with your desired outcome, which is the fruit of your Faith. In other words, if you're seeking financial abundance, you can't hope for financial catastrophe to befall a colleague. Your hoping has a direct impact upon your Faith. Your Faith is seeded in your hope, and hope feeds your Faith. One of the keys to powerful "mountain-moving" Faith is making sure your Faith is well fed by hope. "Your substance of things hoped for" will either bless or curse your Faith. It will either unleash or lock up your Faith.

Since what you hope for plays such an important role in your vision becoming reality, let's take a moment to examine hope as a concept. Hope is expecting God to do what God has promised, regardless of your current situation or human prognosis. Hope is not some pie-in-the-sky notion, denying the painful reality of the moment. Hope, however, does look through that painful reality to the desired outcome, always expecting that outcome to move toward fruition.

The second story about Faith involves hope. Two five-year-olds were placed in two different rooms. One child's room was filled with brand-new toys. The other child's room was filled with manure. Two hours later, each five-year-old was revisited. In the room with the toys, every brand-new item was destroyed practically beyond recognition. But in the room filled with manure, an amazing phenomenon had taken place. The manure had been rearranged and stacked into neat little piles. The five-year-old emerged from the room with manure on her shoes, shirt, and pants.

"Why did you rearrange the manure, and why do you have manure all over your clothes?" she was asked.

"With all that manure in that room, there must be a pony or a horse in there somewhere," she replied. "And I am going to find him!"

Hope refuses to allow a messy, even stinky, situation to hold it down or to restrict its creativity. Hope is the desire for a better world; Faith propels you to walk out on that desire. The only one who can truly restrict your hope, and thus your Faith, is you. The woman with the biscuit on her back didn't have Faith; the five-year-old with manure on her clothing did.

GOOD STEWARDSHIP

The second ingredient in God's mathematics is just as important as Faith: stewardship. God owns the world and all its bounty. We are stewards—managers or caretakers—of God's possessions. In order to be more faithful of our blessings, we must learn to use wisely what the Provider has given us. We must be a good steward of whatever we've been given. Because whatever we've been given has the ability to multiply.

> *Now, the Passover, a feast of the Jews, was near. Then, Jesus lifted up his eyes and seeing a great multitude coming toward him, said to Philip, "Where shall we buy bread that these may eat?" But this he said to test him, for he himself knew what he would do. Philip answered him, "Two hundred denari worth of bread is not sufficient for them, that every one of them may have a little." One of his disciples, Andrew, Simon Peter's brother, said to him, "There is a lad here who has five barley loaves and two small fish, but what are they among so many?" Then, Jesus said, "Make the people sit down." Now, there was so much grass in the place, so the men sat down in number about 5,000, and Jesus took the loaves and when had given thanks he distributed them to the disciples and the disciples to those sitting down and likewise of the fish, as much as they wanted. So when they were filled, he said to his disciples, "Gather up the fragments that remain so that nothing is lost."*
> —JOHN 6:4–12

One of the main ways Jesus taught is through parables. A parable, roughly defined, is a seemingly simple story that carries some greater truth or meaning. In this way, each parable had two parts: the surface story and the deeper truth. "The marrow of a parable is different from the promise of its surface, and like as gold is sought for in the earth, the kernel in a nut, and the hidden fruit in the prickly covering of chestnuts, so in parables we must search more deeply after the divine meaning," said one early Church father.

The Parables of Jesus focused on children, parties, feasts, wineskins, orchards, and most frequently, money. More than half of Jesus' parables had to do with money. The famous story of the loaves and fishes in John 6:4–12 has the qualities of a parable. The seemingly simple story belies a greater kernel of truth: the second principle in God's mathematics.

Let's study the story.

After Jesus fed the people with the word of God, they were hungry physically. Being concerned about the whole person, and not just the spiritual side, Jesus said, "Well, it's time to feed 'em some food." He had 200 denari—probably less than $50—and 5,000 men, not including women and children, to feed. Can't you hear the naysayers? "How on earth are you going to feed five thousand men with fifty dollars' worth of groceries?"

Somebody reading this book right now is in a similar situation financially. You know who you are. You've got so many critical needs for money but so few sources. You've got people baying for cash on all sides, but nothing to give back to them. Just as Jesus had 5,000 men to feed with $50, you've got a life to feed on pitifully too few dollars.

What did Jesus do? Just what you've got to do if you're going to come up with some winning numbers in God's mathematics:

1. Assess your situation.

In the Bible, Jesus says to Philip, "Where shall we buy bread that these may eat?" That's the fifth verse. In other words, *Let's see what we have.*

It makes such good sense. But so many of us don't really know what we have! We're so busy trying to rob Peter to pay Paul, we never take time out for self-inventory, for self-examination. We're too busy working 21.5 part-time jobs. We're so busy rippin' and runnin', we've yet to sit down and systematically list our assets and our liabilities. We don't know what we already have emotionally and spiritually and how that wealth might enrich us economically.

"How are you doing?" you ask these folks too busy for self-inventory and self-examination.

"I'm broke," they'll reply.

It's a sign, a symptom, of trouble at the core. You didn't ask this person for an analysis of their financial situation. You asked them how they're doing! But they've so entangled their self-worth in their financial situation, they're unable to separate wallet from soul.

If you think money can buy automatic happiness, consider this newspaper story from the August 16, 1961, edition of the *Louisville Courier* that Robert Sardello quoted in his book *Facing the World with Soul:*

> More than $150,000 in cash and securities was unearthed Tuesday in the Yorkville district apartment of an eccentric who piled about him the accumulated trash and tokens of year upon year of solitude. Amid the debris were faded reminders of life in New York half a century ago.
>
> George Aichele, 73, was found dead Monday of natural causes. It took police all night to ferret out and

count $47,000 in cash in the five-room flat, including $500 and $1,000 bills casually tucked amid rubbish.

More than 80 bank books were also turned up, noting deposits of more than $112,000. Some of the deposits, of only $10, were made, a friend said, because Aichele coveted the minor gifts with which banks encouraged new depositors.

Aichele was an incredible hoarder. He even wrapped a single penny and tucked it away with a notation he had found it outside his 66th Street apartment.

"In the living room the junk was piled 5 feet high," said Patrolman James Pyne, first to enter the apartment after Aichele's lawyer missed the old bachelor for many days. There were razors and blades, newspapers and magazines dated at the turn of the century, unopened cases of liquor, phonograph records, thousands of packs of safety matches, dozens of wedding bands and diamond rings, a carton of more than 100 harmonicas, a bird cage, a zither. Aichele was a recluse as far as his home was concerned. No one but himself was known to have set foot inside it since a brother with whom he lived died 13 years ago. This brother, John, presumably took part in the hoarding, since much of the trash accumulated antedated his death in 1947. Another brother, Henry, a bank executive, died in 1956, also amid rubbish accumulated in his home. It took six months to clear it out. The brothers inherited money from their father, Charles, who made a fortune in Manhattan real estate.

Just as the character described in the *Louisville Courier* hoarded his possessions, many of us unconsciously hoard our God-given talents by constantly focusing on our weaknesses. You can spend a lifetime trying to perfect your weaknesses. You'll have weaknesses with you always. The champions among us know their strengths and build upon them. The chumps get so tangled up in their weaknesses they never have a chance to examine their strengths. It's just as sinful to live beneath your means as it is to live above them.

Don't ever doubt that you have strengths. Satan will attempt to blind your eyes and plug your ears to your own ability and to God's awesome power. God has blessed you with strengths. It's your duty to know what they are. Far too many folks go to their grave attempting to perfect their weaknesses and never maximizing their strengths. You've got to discover what the Bible calls your gifts and talents. Stop majoring in the minor. Satan will tempt you to spend your precious time and energy on useless projects. If it's not your gift and if it's not your talent, then you're wasting your precious time. It's like putting fertilizer on concrete and expecting grass to grow. Get a grip! Ask yourself, *What are my gifts? What are my talents? What are my God-given competencies?* Assess your situation. Don't spend a lifetime perfecting imperfection. Focus in on what your purpose is in your life.

Find out what you have.

When we took an inventory of what we had in our community, what resources might help us raise the $2.6 million, which would rapidly escalate to more than $5 million, to build The Power Center, our assets were few. But our allies were many. We were blessed with the resource of people. We decided our members would be the source of our strength. We wouldn't hold fish fries or potluck dinners or bake sales. I'm not saying that fish fries, potluck dinners, and bake sales aren't viable fundraising techniques for some community-based organizations. In our case though, implementing the strategy of fish fries, potluck dinners, and bake sales would have been God's secondary, as opposed to primary, strategy for raising funds. God was calling us to help ourselves, to raise money from the very people who would share in the glory of The Power Center. This realization gave us the power of self-sufficiency. We suddenly found ourselves surrounded by folks who were willing to make an indelibly Divine difference in someone else's life by investing in a community project.

Take an inventory of your own situation. Maximize the resourcefulness of your present environment.

2. Sit down!

The next thing, after Jesus and the Disciples had taken an inventory of what they had, Jesus said, "Make the people sit down!" Right there, in the tenth verse, we see the 5,000 hungry men. If the offering wasn't organized, if the bread had just been thrown out to them, then the strong men would've elbowed out the weak men, women, and children and would have eaten up all the fish and the bread.

In sitting down, you have a chance to logically arrange your priorities. I think that's what Jesus meant in John 6:10 when he said, "Have the people sit down." I love this as a metaphor: sit down! All this fussing and fighting, mumbling and grumbling—sit down! All this back stabbing and backbiting—sit down! All this finger pointing and he-said, she-said, you-said, they-said—*sit down!* All this running here and yonder, trying to show up and show off, *sit your Humpty-Dumpty backside down!*

Some folks have demons keeping them running day and night! You need to say to those demons, Sit down. Hatred, sit down. Stinginess, sit down. Envy, sit down. Small-mindedness, sit down. Ageism, sit down. Racism, sit down. Sexism, sit down. Self-centeredness, sit down. Doubt, sit down. Depression, sit down. Poverty, sit down. We are in a war against evil. Don't let any kind of thought inhabit your consciousness. Take evil thoughts into captivity. Take authority! Take an assessment! Sit down!

What are your priorities?

Take a moment now and write them down.

There are two major priorities that you are going to have to face if you're going to walk, instead of stumble, into the twenty-first century. They're forever bound together: self-esteem and economics. In the African-American community, we spend up to $400 billion annually. If you were to isolate the dollars spent by African Americans in America, it would perhaps be the eighth-greatest-spending nation in the world. By necessity or compulsion, we currently spend more money than we earn! Our marginal propensity to consume, as economists call it, is high. Make no mistake about it: this is a trick of the devil. There are no banks in most African-American neighborhoods, no savings institutions, no S&Ls. Still, we are what the economists call conspicuous consumers.

As a nation, America is currently experiencing the highest per capita credit-card debt in the history of America. Our country's marginal propensity to consume has risen appreciably over the past five years. We've become a nation of spenders, not savers. But the higher your personal savings rate, the stronger your economic prowess.

We cannot hold anybody else responsible for our own habits. We have to take charge; we have to take an assessment. We spend too much money on stuff we don't need, trying to impress people who don't even like us! We need to sit down. We need to arrange our priorities. The stuff you think you want, can it wait until next year, next quarter, next budget?

In Luke 14:28, it's written, "Will he not first sit down and estimate the cost to see if he has enough money to complete it? For if he lays the foundation and is not able to finish it, everyone will ridicule him saying, 'This fellow began to build and was not able to finish.'"

When the board of The Power Center sat down to arrange our

priorities, these priorities stretched across the page in logical formation. Soon, we developed a strategy, a creed, a vocabulary that defined our mission.

Here are a few of the phrases that guided us:

Impossible just means it may take a little longer. When somebody tells you something that is "impossible," take it as a sign that you're on to something worthwhile. Realize that nothing is impossible when it is ordained by God. The truly great accomplishments in life were all once impossible. Realize it just means that it takes a little longer.

Finance yourself. Whether you're financing a new life or a new project, funding is critical. But try not to let yourself become beholden to anyone or anything for money. In our case, we had banks willing to lend us the $2 million for our Power Center. But by issuing our own bonds bought by our own members, we became our own financier, as opposed to the bank. We never had to do those things that usually have to be done to meet other people's expectations. We never had to sell our soul; our Power Center was self-sufficient.

(I'm not saying you shouldn't borrow to finance your Vision. When you borrow, however, be careful not to leverage your soul. Yes, you can take a mortgage out on your home—just make sure your budget can take the monthly payments. And if you need to borrow to get through school, then have a plan to pay back what you owe so you can eventually reap *all* the rewards of your hard-earned education. But whatever you do, *don't* borrow carelessly or thoughtlessly—for instance, because you don't know how much you've got in the bank or because you don't want to wait until next month's paycheck for that outfit, or those sneakers, or that new stereo you covet. Count the cost!)

Learn to live in limbo. When you're growing, you're going to have times when you won't know what tomorrow will bring. Learn to live in limbo, instead of abandoning your path out of fear of the uncertain. That's the essence of the Faith Walk—the limbo, the uncertainty, the unknowing. You must learn to do what you can do with what you've been shown and let God handle the unseen and as-yet-unknown. Learn to live in limbo without being anxious about what has not happened yet.

Everything must make sense—and cents. Whether you're running a family or a business, write these words in block letters above your desk: Everything Must Cash Flow. Life runs on emotions, but you have to back it up with dollars and cents. Your financial life has to make cents!—not just sense.

God will show you just enough to keep you productive. You are on a wondrous mission. If you knew everything up front—all of the slipups and pratfalls and escalating costs—you wouldn't begin the walk. You'd be paralyzed. If we'd known that it would take us almost three years to get The Power Center up and running, that the final price tag would be over $5 million, when we thought it would be $2.6 and take us eighteen months, we would have been paralyzed. It would've seemed too big to begin. But God showed us just enough to keep us moving. As we moved, we remembered the old adage about the elephant: How do you eat an elephant? Bite by bite. You have to balance planning with Faith, especially with the obstacles that we had. God gave us just enough to keep us productive.

Unwritten were the wiles of the devil, which haunted us at practically every turn, especially through the guise of negativity. When we tried to raise the money and started the fundraising, some people wondered, "Why?" One of Satan's most effective strategies in sowing discord is through others. In our case, as we set out on our mission of enlisting donations from the membership, we would hear period-

ically comments like "Why are you doing that?" Satan tried to dis-
courage us from getting people to give to the project.

The other way Satan tried to dismantle the project is through
what we began to call the "something else's." We always needed
more money, or movement, than we had. You'll be at point A,
when you need to be at point B. Consider this a testing of your
Faith. God wants to see how you'll handle certain circumstances.
Through it all, we believed—we trusted that the Lord knew what
we needed and that He would provide.

3. Give thanks to God.

Once Jesus received the loaves and fishes, He gave the food to His
disciples and the disciples gave it to the people. He was always or-
ganizing, always prioritizing, always working with a procedure—
process and orderliness. Then, when the work was done, the final
yet crucial step was giving thanks to the Supplier of the blessings.
Once you assess your situation and arrange your priorities, you
must, as the Bible says, thank God. In John, Jesus gave thanks for
the miraculous multiplication of the fish and the loaves. We must
thank God for the blessings He has bestowed upon us. As the late
Reverend James Cleveland once sang, "'Thank you' makes room
for more."

So the Stewardship process has three legs: Assess, arrange, adore.

Assess Your Situation

Arrange Your Priorities

Adore God in All Ways

In other words, give God some praise. You may not have what
you used to have. But you can still praise God. You may not have

CREATING WEALTH GOD'S WAY

what you think you ought to have. But you can still praise God. This is an integral part of God's mathematics. Without praise, you will not consistently receive God's miraculous multiplication process. If you don't give God the praise, then the miraculous multiplication process is inhibited. We're going to get to that miraculous multiplication process in a moment. You'll discover that it is a multiplication process with better odds than you'd get in Las Vegas, much less the lottery. I'm talking about everything you give to God coming back to you tenfold. But first let's focus in on praise.

Now, I can hear somebody reading this book saying, *"Things are so tough for me right now, Kirbyjon, I can't praise anybody."*

Praise, in the form of prayer, was pivotal to the success of building our Power Center. What else did we have? Here we were, the members of a Church, which had been close to closing a decade before, now facing down a financial challenge nothing short of audacious: to raise $1.2 million and float a bond of an equal amount in twenty-four months. As I've said, we weren't an army of experts. Our Building Committee was five downright amateurs when it came to constructing a multimillion-dollar building. Our strength was in our Faith. We believed. We met regularly for two years, confident of both our Faith in God and the support of the congregation. We were merely the instrument through which God's blessings could flow.

At this juncture, the emphasis my wife Suzette had been placing on the power of corporate prayer in the life of the Church showed up—big-time. We prayed. Lord, did we pray. At every meeting of our Pyramid Community Development Corporation, we'd ask for God's guidance in the decisions that we needed to make. We prayed that God would send us the people we needed to get the job done and that the Lord would continue to encourage us to be good stewards of the blessings we'd already received. And each time we needed something or someone—whether it was a contractor, supplier, or contact—the

Lord would place someone in our path who would provide whatever we needed. We needed a kitchen, but we didn't have the millions necessary to build a professional restaurant kitchen. God sent us Harris Pappas, one of the owners of the Pappas family chain of restaurants, headquartered in Houston. Pappas's architects drew up the plans for our kitchens, designed them, and donated all of the equipment. Thank God for Pappas Restaurants!

As the project began gaining steam, we conducted prayer walks through the vacant old building: We pulled our congregation together one morning at 7 and we formed a human circle of five hundred people around that dilapidated building and prayed and prayed and prayed. Try it: gather your family around something you're dreaming of doing and pray on it. You'll discover something awesome, energizing, and galvanizing.

We needed funding. We prayed. We had staffing issues, tenant issues popping up. We prayed. When construction was half-finished, we encircled it and prayed, always dedicating the building back to the Lord. We'd pray on one subject, then revolve collectively in a human chain around the building, and then pray on something else.

We never had a doubt that God heard our prayers. When hostilities or negative undercurrents arose, we had what we called Emergency Prayer. Usually, our prayers would be answered in a way that demanded our involvement. That's one way God blesses. If you are praying for your wayward child, God will do something in your life that will involve your doing something to change your wayward child. When God starts working for the community, He will work through the people who have been praying for the community. When you pray for your nation, don't think that you won't have a job to do when God answers your prayer—God's blessings will involve some effort from you. You're going to have to work to fulfill the answer to the prayer. You can't just pray for abundance and expect to win the lottery, or expect the anonymous man from that old TV show *The Millionaire* to show up on your doorstep with a check.

When you pray, be prepared to back up your prayer with *action.*

GIVING

But I say, he which soweth sparingly shall reap also sparingly. And he which soweth bountifully shall reap also bountifully. Every man according as he purposed in his heart, so let him give. Not begrudgingly or of necessity. For the Lord loves a cheerful giver and God is able to make all grace abound toward you that ye always having all sufficiency in all things may abound to every good work. As it is written, he has disbursed abroad, he has given to the poor his righteousness reigneth forever. . . . Thanksgiving to God.
—2 CORINTHIANS 9:6–11

Once you begin looking at the world as belonging to God, you'll be amazed at how you can position yourself to be blessed. Blessings flow as freely and as powerfully as water through a garden hose. If you're not getting your "fair share" of blessings, it's very likely that you've got a glitch in your hose.

I learned an illuminating dramatization from Bishop T. D. Jakes in Dallas, which I passed on to my congregation. Let me show it to you. On the pulpit, I shake out the cord on the microphone and say to the congregation, "Pretend this is a water hose."

Now, a water hose and a bank account have more in common than you might initially think. Through a water hose flows current; through a bank account flows currency. But both can fall prey to blockages if the operator of either the hose or the bank account is not vigilant in operating the instrument that delivers either current or currency.

Through the hose, I tell my congregation from the pulpit,

flows God's wondrous blessings, roaring through that hose for each of us as fast as it would for a fireman battling a three-alarm blaze. The Lord intends for us to get *every drop* of water that He delivers through that hose. But some of us do things, intentionally and unintentionally, to cause a *glitch* in our hose.

I twist the microphone wire.

"When you do something that is not of God and you don't repent about it, you get a glitch in your hose," I say.

I twist the microphone wire again.

"When God blesses you with a thirty-thousand-dollar-a-year job and you capriciously spend thirty-five-thousand, you have a glitch in your hose," I say. "When God forgives you but you don't forgive somebody else, you have a glitch in your hose. When God has given you His blessings but you sit on them, sprawled out in front of the TV, when you know, deep down, God intends for you to represent the Kingdom and help someone else, you have a glitch in your hose. When God is prospering your business, but you treat your employees unfairly, you have a glitch in your hose."

I twist the wire again and again until it is knotted with glitches.

"Now, not only is your hose shorter than it was before, so you can't get everything God intended you to have because it's all tied up in your glitches," I say, "but then, you have the audacity to get mad at God. You need to get mad at the devil and reprioritize your life!"

God has promised you power, abundance, and good success. He has promised you prosperity, right there in the book of Joshua. But every privilege promised by God comes with a responsibility. To get your fair share of blessings, you should begin to untangle the glitches that have dammed up your hose.

How? First, realize that God is both the water and the hose, the Supply and the Supplier. And since God is the Supply and the Supplier of all things, then it makes sense to do what the Supplier says to do about His economics. Satan is the temporary prince of this society. But there will never be more than one king. God still expects and looks for His people to be good and faithful, even during trying times.

Ever notice how God blesses? Every day God just pours out one blessing after another. When we're good, God blesses. When we're bad, God blesses. When we're right, God blesses. When we're wrong, God blesses. He's just a blessing God. By grace, the Lord will pour out blessings that you won't even have room for—if you're faithful. Too many of us mess up our blessings. We drop our stuff on the floor. We make a mess out of God's blessings. Every time we fail to give or live according to God's Way and Word, we gnaw away at our capacity for blessedness. Position yourself to be blessed!

GOD'S MIRACULOUS
MULTIPLICATION PROCESS

Okay, now let's discuss perhaps the greatest investment system known to mankind, God's awesome formula for creating abundance. Allow me to reveal it to you in the same way I first discussed it with the congregation at Windsor Village. We were in the old sanctuary, maybe 110 of us, when I walked down the aisle with a blackboard and a piece of chalk.

I drew a pie on the blackboard and told the congregation that the pie represented our personal wealth, of which we are stewards for God.

"If the world and its bounty belong to God, and what we give back to Him is our 'rent' for occupying space on earth, how much rent does God expect from us?" I asked the congregation.

There was a collective pause before the congregation began throwing out figures.

"No," I said. "All God requires of us is ten percent. You should

save ten percent and then live on eighty percent. How many corpo-
rations do you know that would offer you a ninety percent return
on a meager ten percent investment?"

Some members laughed, but it's true. In tithing your time,
your money, and your talent, the suggested model for spiritual success is 10 percent to God, 10 percent to savings, and 80 percent for
living. If you can redesign your personal finances along these ra-
tios, you'll be amazed at what will come back to you. The 10 percent is not a random figure; the word *tithe* actually comes from a
Greek word meaning "a tenth of the whole." In Biblical days, God
actually commanded the Israelites to give 10 percent of their income to their religious temples. It works for us today!

One member of our congregation, Pam Calip, and her husband watched miracles firsthand when she began to tithe 10 percent of their time, talent, and total income to God.

"When we started to tithe, we were in need of a car. Not only
were we able to get the car, it was provided in such a way that it was
not only timely but very affordable," says Pam. "Another time, my
husband was out of work for two years, and we had enough
money—he got a lump sum when the company laid him off and
we tithed it immediately (ten percent of it)—and we had enough
money to live on. If he had not worked for four years, we would
have never missed a bill. One portion of being a good steward was
to use your gifts, times, talents . . . untold things happen."

She discovered that when she gives freely to others, God
blesses. But sometimes the blessings aren't meant to stay with you
but flow through you. "Somebody came up and said, 'The Lord
just told me to give you this.' And it was a hundred-dollar bill. We
prayed on it, and thought the blessing was flowing through us. A
little later, a woman came up to us, she had been evicted from her
apartment and had some other things going on in her life. She had
a job, but she hadn't been in it long enough for her to put gas in her

car. As she spoke, I knew the money was for her. It had come through me, but it was for her. Tithing makes you a better assessor of people's needs."

At Windsor Village, we started a personal finance ministry, studying the excellent book *Managing Your Money God's Way,* by Larry Burkett, which also relies on the 80–10–10 principle. The members of the ministry were amazed at their returns.

"I found that every time I increased my giving, I received more: whether it was a raise in my job or unexpected money in the mail because I overpaid something," remembers Genora Boykins. "Every time I was faithful in giving, I'd receive. I also learned that the tithing wasn't just in money, but time. Some people would give money but not time. I have been rewarded because of that. I've been given opportunities beyond what I'd ever expected. I've never done anything so that I could be lifted up. Some people just desire or thirst after authority or power. That's never been anything I've desired. But I've found myself in a leadership position, and I trust that God placed me there because of my obedience and my time."

Another member of Windsor Village, Russell Jackson, the owner of his own research-evaluation company, recently discovered the wonders of giving to God. In the last year, he's increased his tithes of both time and money to 10 percent of his gross income. "As my Faith in God increased, I felt more comfortable in tithing, knowing that whatever I tithed would be returned manyfold," he says. "Within the past two years, I've begun to pray over my business. I've grown from a three-person operation to having a permanent staff of ten and more than forty people working in contract roles around the country. Recently, I made a commitment to an altar call for an offering. Thirty men were asked to each 'seed' $198 to the prayer institute. When I went up to the altar to give my donation, the guest pastor leading the revival looked at me and said, 'How much do you want to make out of your business this year?' I replied, 'One million dollars,' and he said, 'You're going to have that and more.'

"The next Tuesday, I had to make a presentation for a business project in Washington, D.C. I was competing against four different firms. On the Sunday night I made the $198 offering, I suddenly got an incredible insight that undoubtedly came from God in terms of how I needed to present my capabilities in Washington. When I got to Washington, I was told that everybody else had come with *teams* of people; they were surprised that I had come alone. But I was on my game. That was on a Tuesday. Back in Houston the next Monday, I got a call saying, 'You won the competition. The value of that project is going to be about a million dollars.'"

Adds Jackson, "Those are the kinds of blessings with which I've been bestowed. Since we've made a commitment to give both time and money to God, my family and I have just reaped blessings upon blessings."

Don't get me wrong. God is not a slot machine, your personal waiter, or your bell boy. Russell Jackson does not tithe so that God will "pay him back." He tithes because he loves and trusts God enough to step out on Faith. When you tithe, you release inhibiting shackles, becoming free to be more sensitive to God's leadership. Tithing is not restricted to any denomination or belief system. Every community has its own concept of giving. Give freely. Give of your money, your time, your teachings, your leadership, your energy. Give at least 10 percent of yourself.

Some folk view tithing as an Old Testament principle for Old Testament days. I invite you, however, to prayerfully consider stepping up to the tithe—or at least move in that direction—as a testimony of your love for your Lord and your community. God is not a slot machine, but God does reward faithfulness. Give unto the Lord and he will give back to you, pressed down, shaken together and running over.

THE POWER OF TWO HOURS

Frequently, God's miraculous multiplication works when we invest our time in noble causes. This was the case of Rod Bailey, a member of Windsor Village, who almost flunked out of high school, until he learned how to invest in himself and thus make a future investment to God. Rod had promise, but he wouldn't crack a book! When his teachers would put him in study hall, he'd fall asleep. When his parents would lock him in his room, demanding that he study, he'd drift off into daydream.

Then, he learned the Power of Two Hours.

That's right, two hours. That's all. Whether it's launching a new business endeavor, learning a new skill, or studying, start with two hours—and watch how rapidly those two hours multiply. Rod Bailey wasn't ready to devote his life to studying, an image that, with their stern directives, his teachers and parents had conjured up. But he could sacrifice two hours.

Something amazing happened to this young man. Within six weeks, his grades had gone from failing to a B average. Shortly afterward, he graduated from high school with honors, his grade-point average among the top 25 percent of his class. Now, having graduated with honors from college, he is successful financially in his job at the Fort Bend Council of Economic Development and spiritually in his dedication to God.

Two hours—that's all. A meager investment of time can grow into a new life.

Donate your time, energy, and talents to both God and yourself. You'll be amazed at what comes back to you. How you invest your time and money is an unswervingly clear indicator of what you deem important. Your checkbook and daily calendar speak much louder than your verbal declarations of service.

Managing Your Money God's Way

"Therefore I tell you, do not worry about your life, what you will eat or drink, or about your body, what you will wear. Is not life more important than food and the body more important than clothes? . . . But seek first His kingdom and His righteousness and all these things will be added or given to you, as well."
—Matthew 6:25–33

Once God blesses you with abundance, the Lord expects you to be a good steward of God's gifts. A few years back, prior to their becoming clergy, Rudy and Juanita Rasmus presented an empowering fifteen-week Bible-study seminar at Windsor Village. We called it "Money Honey/Honey Hush," named for the old colloquialism reflecting many people's intimidation when it comes to even talking about finances. These people, usually in debt, are absolutely terrified to open the door on the haunted house of their finances.

Here are a few key principles the Bible-study group examined:

1. *Change Your Attitude.* Understand that much of your attitude about money has been inherited from your parents. Take an attitude inventory. Are you an impulse spender? A hoarder? A shopaholic? A clothes addict? Are you spending to get other needs met? Once you understand your attitude toward money, ask yourself, "Is my attitude Bible- or marketplace-based?" In the book *In Search of Significance,* author Robert McGee says most of us operate out of four basic attitudes: performance (buying as reward); approval (buying to feel worthy); blame (buying to overcome perceived negativity); shame (buying as compensation for low self-esteem). If you fit into one or more of these categories, acknowledge it, confess it, and change. Remember the words of the late Moms Mabley: "If you always do what you've always done, you'll get what you've always gotten."

2. *Establish a Budget*: If you're going to honor the Lord, I encourage you to give according to Malachi 3:10, "Bring ye all the tithes to the storehouse." It's been written that a Christian requires two conversions: first the heart, then the pocketbook. Writing down your monthly income and expenditures is a crucial first step. How do you know where you're going to go if you don't know where you already are? Most people are intimidated by the process of writing down what they spend. But that simple step is the genesis of accountability.

3. *Curb Impulse Spending*. Cut up your credit cards! A member of the Bible-study group had twenty-five credit cards, all charged to the max. She brought them all to the church and we baked them on a cookie sheet and gave out them out as trophies symbolizing her liberation over debt. There is an underlying motive to your spending. It's your duty to determine what it is. One of the things we've discovered about impulse buying is that it stems from unmet needs, most frequently a need for intimacy. We think we can buy ourselves out of loneliness and unworthiness. And the market is always open. I've heard we're exposed to more than 70,000 commercials per day, from radio, TV, and the subliminal messages on people's blue jeans, T-shirts, and coffee cups. We're bombarded by messages that say, "If you want to change, spend, buy, charge!" But God doesn't care what kind of car you drive or the watch on your wrist. Discover why you spend and you'll discover a lot of what you are lacking spiritually.

4. *Saving*. After you give one-tenth to God, give at least 10 percent to your savings account, which can be used as an emergency fund. God hasn't called you to be in want. Part of the provision for your needs must be a routine savings plan. You must systematically provide for your future: continuing education, a career change, or unexpected investment opportunities that God might send your way. (And I'm not talking about get-rich-quick schemes!) The Word says that a wise man will leave an inheritance to his children's children. We're talking about leaving an inheritance not only of money, but the integrity you attach

to money. Would you want to leave your children the inheritance of your spending patterns? (Past-due notices, pink slips, credit-card delinquency bills?) Do you want to teach them to live paycheck-to-paycheck or to embark upon a lifetime of good, sound stewardship?

5. *Get Rid of What You Don't Need!* Remember, excess equates to waste. Whatever you have that you're not using, you're wasting. As it is written in Luke 12:33, "Sell what you have and make an offering to those who are in need." Always remember, this is not our stuff, this is God's stuff! Identify the things you're hanging on to, then sell, give away, or throw out the things that are hindering you financially. For instance, how about the boat you use twice a year but make twelve excruciating payments for annually? Sell it or rent it out to generate extra income for debt reduction.

6. *Free Yourself of Excess Debt.* Careless debt creates bondage. I'm talking particularly about credit-card interest rates, unpaid loans, and the pileup of unnecessary charge cards. It's been estimated that a substantial percentage of people in mental hospitals got there, in part, because of the stress and anxiety caused by improper money management. Anxiety takes you nowhere—but down. As it's written in Matthew 6:27, "Which of you by worrying can add one cubit to his stature?"

7. *Learn How to Be Content with What You Have.* I'm not suggesting you not set financial goals. What I am saying is develop an attitude of gratitude, being thankful at every stage for what you already have. In Philippians 4–11, when Paul was in prison, he says, "I have learned in whatever state I am, to be content."

8. *Above All, Have Faith.* "Well done, good and faithful servant; you were faithful over a few things, I will make you ruler over many things," Jesus tells his disciples in Matthew 25:21. The root of both the word *disciple* and the word *discipline* are the same. God is calling you to be a disciplined disciple over your finances. In this way, you can become truly rich.

You Can Breathe New Life
into Dried Bones

*And he said unto me, "Son of man, can these bones live?" And I
answered, "O Lord God, thou knowest." Again he said to me,
"Prophesy upon these bones, and say unto them, O ye dry bones,
hear the word of the Lord. Thus saith the Lord God unto these
bones; Behold, I will cause breath to enter into you, and ye shall
live: and I will lay sinews upon you, and will bring up flesh upon
you, and cover you with skin, and put breath in you, and ye shall
live; and ye shall know that I am the Lord."*

—EZEKIEL 37:3–6

It is one of the Bible's most dramatic and miraculous spectacles.
There stands the seraphic Ezekiel, whose very name means "God
will strengthen," in a valley of dried human bones, such a plain of
death and destruction that the dried bones are strewn as thick as a
blizzard's snowfall, bleached white by long exposure to the sun.
The story is, of course, a parable: the bones are representative of
the destitute spiritual condition of the sinful Israelites. Could these
bones live? Certainly not. But God shows Ezekiel that "what is impossible with man is possible with God" by demonstrating His
power in that valley.

"Prophesy upon these bones," God commands, and when
Ezekiel does as ordered, the earth begins to shake. "As I prophesied
there was a noise, and behold a shaking, and the bones came together, bone to his bone . . . the sinews and the flesh came up upon
them, and the skin covered them above," says Ezekiel.

The bones had no breath, of course, but God asks Ezekiel to
prophesy upon the wind, "and the breath came into them, and they
lived, and stood up upon their feet, an exceeding great army."

The story is God's way of showing the Israelites that just as

God created humanity from dust, so has the Lord commanded Israel to realize that the Almighty God could open their graves, symbolic of the hope that had died within them, and bring them into the kingdom of Israel.

The message for today's times? God can breathe life into what has dried up, or died, within us. We can take the dry bones of our existence, no matter how bleached by the forces of evil, and make them live anew. We can create armies of strength from plains of frailty. God's power is able!

We are able to do so because God empowers it to be so. God empowers us, then we can empower others. In the case of our congregation, the dry bones was that asbestos-filled building that we had been deeded and into which we would breathe new life by taking responsibility for ourselves and our community. *Responsibility*. It's an integral component for economic abundance. If we are to rise above the dried bones of our past, we must learn to empower ourselves for the future. Empowerment is the purpose of The Power Center. Our mission statement comes from Isaiah 61:3: "They shall repair the ruined cities and restore what has long lain desolate." But empowerment was also the propulsion that got The Power Center built. In order to best serve God, we must learn to use what we have been given. You cannot expect your employers, schools, systems, and governments to supply your needs. You must take responsibility and move forward, breathing new life into those dry bones.

Once you breathe that first breath, a miracle will take place. Others will rise to help you. We discovered this firsthand in developing the once asbestos-filled buildings—the dry bones of another community facing economic hard times—into The Power Center. As a result of the generosity of Fiesta, Inc., which donated the land, the members of the Windsor Village Church family and friends, with the help of private donations, have been able to create more than 280 new jobs in a building that was an eyesore only three short years ago.

How did we do it?

By practicing the equation for God's mathematics:

Faith + Good Stewardship + Giving = Abundance

All three components require taking responsibility.

We wanted more people to be employed and employable and have a stronger community economic base. We wanted more people to own their own homes and take more pride in both their community and themselves. We wanted to raise the level of how people in our community felt about themselves. We wanted to address the tangible needs of our community, as well as give our people a symbol of hope.

So we took responsibility for the situation. We took responsibility for a dilapidated rat-infested eyesore, a vacated Kmart building, consisting of 104,000 square feet. We invested about $600,000 of the Church Family members' hard-earned money, acquired a grant from the U.S. government, secured some foundation support and borrowed the balance, and now we have renovated that old Kmart building into what is today a paradigm of how private enterprise and nonprofit entities can and, I believe, *must* come together in order to make an indelibly Divine difference, impacting the complicated social/economic issues of the twenty-first century.

Our Faith—and most important, our Faith Walk—has paid off in ways we couldn't have imagined. One step, no matter how feeble in the beginning, led us to a wondrous destination. I invite you to visit The Power Center. We have a Chase Bank of Texas branch, the first bank branch in our community. The traditional interpretation of data indicated that that community would not and could not support a bank branch. Now it can. Chase Bank of Texas, formerly Texas Commerce Bank, led by then-chairman and CEO Marc Shapiro, had Faith in the purpose of The Power Center.

We took responsibility for the educational needs of the community by creating the Imani School for Children and the Houston Community College Business Technology Center for adults in The Power Center. We took responsibility for our community's medical welfare by creating a clinic in The Power Center to meet the medical needs of the community. We took responsibility for developing entrepreneurship by creating twenty-seven business suites and commercial lease space. We have the fourth-largest banquet facility in the city of Houston. We can seat 1,200 people for a sit-down dinner, 2,200 people auditorium-style. What began as a mere thought for a vacant, non–income-producing eyesore has become a vital multi-million community-based blessing that is producing more than 260 new jobs and will pump $28.7 million into the local community over the next three years.

The Bible says, If you don't work, then you shouldn't eat. We wanted to create jobs and to create opportunities and build hope and inspiration among the members of the community. God has blessed the Vision to become a premier example of how "the Word becomes flesh and dwells among us."

I thank God for The Power Center. Recognizing God as its source, our congregation took responsibility for those blessings of the Lord. As it says in the Bible, "Faith without works is dead."

LEARN HOW TO ASK!

One final point about God's mathematics: when your business gives God the glory and meets the needs of people, then do not be afraid to ask for money! If you don't ask for it, you'll never get it. I learned this firsthand when I went to Evander Holyfield, soon to become the three-time heavyweight boxing champion of the world, to ask him for . . . money. Evander belongs to a Church in Atlanta, but when he trains in Houston and is in the city on weekends, he attends Windsor Village.

One day before one of his fights with Buster Douglas, I called him and said, "Evander, I want to pick you up and show you something." I picked him up and drove him over to The Power Center.

"Evander, the Lord is leading us to build a Prayer Center, which will be open twenty-five hours a day, eight days a week," I said, as we looked over the land. "Always available for folks to come and pray."

I looked the champion in the eye and I'm not ashamed to tell you, my old speech impediment returned. I think I actually began to stutter.

"Evander, we've got the Vision for a prayer center," I said. "It's going to cost about $1.2 million. Will you pay fffff—for the pppp-rrayer ccccenter?"

I was just about that nervous. See, the devil had tried to persuade me against even asking the man for help. I thought about and prayed on this for months! It took me many months to ask this man for $1.2 million. But then I learned something important: People are never offended if you ask them for more money than they can give. If that upsets them, they're going to be upset if you asked them for $2.67. They're not insulted by the amount. If they're annoyed, it's because they are vexed about something else.

Evander answered with one word: *"Yes!"*

He said *yes!* He said yes so quickly, I did not think he understood my question.

"Baby, how did it go?" asked my wife, Suzette, when I got home. I said, "Well, I'm not real sure."

"Did you ask him for the money?" she asked.

"Yes, of course," I said.

"Well, what did he say?"

"He said okay!" I shouted.

I tell you this story for a simple reason. Most people never get what they want in life, simply for the reason that they do not know how to ask. It's critical that you learn how to ask, first God, then those who have the power to make things happen. Why are some folks so afraid about asking others for assistance? I believe it stems from fear of rejection and low self-esteem. They haven't given themselves *permission* to succeed. Some folk rise to a certain level, then begin to self-destruct. Their competency exceeds their self-esteem. They implode. The list of victims from the daily political, sports, business, and entertainment worlds is endless—they haven't given themselves permission to rise to the next level. They've hit a self-esteem ceiling.

Until you make the decision that you don't care what the messy-minded, evil-intentioned, rinky-dink folks say about you. Until you make that decision, you're wasting your time and your blessings!

Allow me to end this chapter with a passage from the eighth chapter of Deuteronomy, which has a lot to say about recognizing the source of blessings. At this juncture, Moses was basically teaching and instructing the children of Israel, who had recently been delivered from Pharaoh and his army. They were positioned opposite Palestine in the plain of Moab, and Moses was giving them instructions for the road.

> "Therefore, you shall keep the commandments of the Lord, your
> God, to walk in his ways and to fear him. For the Lord your God is
> bringing you into a good land, a land of brooks of water, of foun-
> tains and springs, that flow out of valleys and hills. A land of wheat
> and barley, of figs and vines and pomegranates, a land of olive oil
> and honey. A land in which you will eat bread without scarcity, in
> which you will lack nothing. A land whose stones are iron and out
> of whose hills you can dig brass. When you have eaten and you are

full, then you shall bless the Lord, your God, for the good land that he has given you. Beware that you do not forget the Lord, your God, by not keeping His commandments, his judgments and his statutes, which I command you today. Lest when you have eaten and are full and have built beautiful houses and dwelled in them. And when your herds and your flocks multiply, and your silver and your gold multiply, and all that you have multiplies . . ."

—DEUTERONOMY 8:6–13

In other words, as your Aesop plan gains interest and your stocks option plan continues to earn interest, as your IRA continues to grow, as you continue to climb up the ladder of your job, don't forget the Lord!

"When your heart is lifted up, don't forget the Lord, your God, who brought you out of the land of Egypt, from the house of bondage; who led you through that great and terrible wilderness . . . thou shalt remember the Lord, thy God: for it is He that giveth you power to get wealth . . ."

—DEUTERONOMY 8:14–18

The Lord has already brought us a mighty long way. God has brought us from darkness to light. The Lord has brought somebody from catching the bus to having two cars. God has brought somebody from wearing hand-me-downs to a closet full of new clothes. The Almighty brought somebody from sickness to health. The King of kings sits high but looks low. The same God who brought the Israelites out of the wilderness can deliver you, too. Recognizing the Lord God Almighty as the source of your blessings with your honor, respect, and praise lays the foundation for your twenty-first-century deliverance.

6

God-Blessed Relationships

BACK TO THE GARDEN

And the Lord God caused a deep sleep to fall upon Adam and he slept: and he took one of his ribs, and closed up the flesh thereof; And the rib, which the Lord God had taken from man, made he a woman and brought her unto the man. And Adam said, "This is now bone of my bones, flesh of my flesh: she shall be called Woman because she was taken out of Man." Therefore shall a man leave his father and his mother, and shall cleave unto his wife: and they shall be one flesh.

—GENESIS 2:21–24

IT STARTS OUT SO GLORIOUSLY AND THEN, LIKE A TRAGIC LOVE affair, goes so abysmally wrong. From the Garden of Eden, the Bible descends from an extraordinary epic of creation into a morality tale, a saga of misguided love, a doomed story of betrayal, disobedience, and evil. Once God gives Adam Eve, his "helpmate," to whom Adam voices perhaps the greatest love sonnet ever spoken— "This is now bone of my bones, flesh of my flesh"—we watch their downfall. From the garden paradise from which they are expelled, Adam and Eve bowed to the perils of earth, giving birth to Cain and Abel, the perpetrator and victim of the world's first murder, followed by descendants who eventually succumb to envy, hatred, thievery, mayhem, and eventually, apocalypse.

These days, the story of Adam and Eve still has tremendous resonance: relationships remain the downfall of so many lives. In this chapter, we're going to return to the garden of good, healthy, God-blessed relationships. I've determined that God-blessed relationships take three stages: first a relationship with God, then a relationship with yourself, and finally, a relationship with the other person. But before we get to building relationships in each of these distinct areas, let's first define what a healthy relationship is.

LEARNING TO LOVE YOURSELF

Even in describing the creation of Eve, the Bible offers guidance to optimal relationships. God caused a deep sleep to fall over Adam, and while Adam was asleep, the Lord removed his rib, from which God created woman. While Adam was sleeping, God did not remove the skull from Adam for the woman to lead Adam around all the time. God didn't remove Adam's brain so Eve could boss Adam around, toss Adam to and fro like a volleyball. Neither did God take the bone from Adam's backside for the woman to follow behind the man, like some indentured servant. The bone is not a club for a man to whip his woman with, or a poker for him to prod her with, or a limbo stick for him to constantly goad and challenge her and make her crawl under backwards. The bone that created woman came from the rib cage, the epicenter, out of the middle of the body for man to walk alongside of woman to communicate with her, to confide in her, to console her. The Bible calls Eve Adam's "helpmate." A helpmate walks with you! Trusts you! Talks with you! Listens to you! Is your shield!

At Windsor Village, we do a lot of work on relationships, because without God-blessed relationships, the other aspects of Holistic Salvation have no joy, no glue, no resonance. If you're miserable in your personal life, then how can you embrace and enjoy the bounty of wealth, health, Faith, or spiritual prosperity? When you're married, engaged, or paired with a low-down, lying, cheating individual, then you've sentenced yourself to a dance with the devil.

Normal human beings have the ability to love. It is not uncommon, however, for an individual to love someone but not know *how* to love them. To make bad matters worse, some folk don't even realize that they don't know how to love. My hope is that this chapter will help empower you to love, to learn how to love, to truly know the way to God-blessed relationships.

UNHOLY DESPERATION

Nowadays, Mr. Bennett is Dallas County inmate No. 98024531, a convicted swindler with a decade-long pattern of talking women into bed and out of their money.

—THE DALLAS MORNING NEWS, APRIL 8, 1998

Why are human beings so desperate? Why are we willing to date, bed, cohabitate with, and marry—and in some cases run this cycle over and over again—any Tom, Pat, or Sherri, without first getting to know the object of our Faith, future, and affections? Would you fire a loaded gun into an anonymous crowd? It may be a rough analogy, but that's what many of us do with our so-called love. We think that for love to exist, for love to be real, we have to fire it out into the world. Some of us blast away with our love as randomly as gangsters commit a drive-by shooting; we barely take time to aim, then are forced to spend the rest of our lives suffering for the random persons we've hit. But for love to be real and lasting, we have to first give birth to it *inside.* Before we can truly love another, we have to learn how to love ourselves.

Loving yourself, among other things, includes learning how to identify and meet your own needs. In the Gospel according to

Luke, Chapter 10, a lawyer asks Jesus the following question: "What shall I do to inherit eternal life?" As the answer, Jesus quotes the "dual love commandment": "You shall love the Lord your God with all thy heart, and with all thy soul, and with all thy strength, and with all your mind; and your neighbor as yourself."

Ah! That speaks volumes. Love your neighbor as yourself. Love your spouse as yourself. Love your fiancée as yourself. Do you see the pattern here? It's tough to love others healthily and completely if you do not first love yourself healthily and completely. Too many people do not know how to love themselves. After all, it's not something taught in traditional education. But as a result of this void in their learning process, they either expect to find that love of themselves from others, fail to love others as they need to be loved, or most frequently, both. You are truly living in fairy-tale land if you expect a manifestation of love from someone else when you are unwilling or unable to offer that love to yourself. *Expectation minus reality equals disappointment.*

You must learn to love yourself! You must learn to love yourself in order to establish a healthy foundation for a healthy relationship. Unhealthy individuals create unhealthy relationships. Unhealthy individuals tend to attract unhealthy individuals.

You must learn to love yourself if you ever expect to have a healthy marriage. A husband ought not to have to depend upon his wife to "feel like a man." A wife ought not to have to depend upon her husband to "feel like a woman." Please don't misunderstand. Husbands should strive to make their wives feel like queens; wives should strive to make their husbands feel like kings. Nonetheless, healthy folks are not dependent on someone else to make them feel loved! Expecting your spouse to make you feel like a man or a woman is asking for trouble. This should be the icing on the cake, not the cake itself.

Loving yourself means identifying your needs and learning how to meet those needs. The late Curtis Tutson told the story about a reasonably well to do woman who was determined to grow in self-love. After attending numerous seminars, reading numerous books, and speaking to numerous professional consultants, she remained unfulfilled in her pursuit of consummated self-love. Following the advice of an old friend, she visited an old sage in southern England who was the spitting image of the stereotypical St. Nicholas. Upon greeting the woman, the bearded old man asked her to read a stack of books approximately three feet high. He closed her up in a dark, dreary room that resembled a cave. He shut the door on her and promised to return the next morning.

When the old man returned the following dawn, he asked her whether she had completed her assignment. Before the woman could complete her sentence indicating that she had not read the books, the old man swatted her with a book and gave her another stack of books, two feet taller than the first! Walking out of the dark room, the sage decreed, "Read this stack along with the first stack and I will see you tomorrow morning."

The following day, the old sage returned early and the wicked process repeated itself: another reprimand, another stack of books. On the fourth day, however, a transformation occurred. As the sage lifted his hand to swat the woman for not having completed her assignment, the woman blocked his arm, protecting herself from another blow. At this juncture, the sage smiled and exclaimed joyfully: "Now, you have discovered the essence of self-love."

SUCCESSFULLY SINGLE

No one's happiness but my own is in my power to achieve or destroy.

—AYN RAND

We have been socialized to believe that being single is a period of transition, a time—brief, some hope—for the search, the dance, the game of *Finding a Mate*. We have been raised to believe in the myth of marriage. We hitch our relationship destiny to the poetry of music. We believe in songs with lyrics like "One is the loneliest number," and titles like "Somebody to Love."

I hear it over and over again: the panic of single folks doing that time-worn mating dance. Everywhere they go—whether it's work, Church, dry cleaners, school, or shopping mall—they're thinking, "Is this the one? Is that the one?" If the object of their usually premature affection is halfway dressed up and breathing, they think they can change them, as if marriage is some kind of magical makeover. The spirit of desperation can be ruthless.

I've discovered that most miserable married folk were miserable while they were single. But somewhere along the line, society has taught us to put pressure on single folks. "When are you gonna get married?" they incessantly ask. Satan specializes in creating a false sense of urgency: *"You need to get married!" "You've got to hurry!" "That clock is ticking!"* Whoa! Take a deep breath, exhale, and remember: all true joy comes from the Lord. If you expect to find joy from somebody else, and you have not found joy yourself, you're setting yourself up for heartbreak. You are setting yourself up for a downfall. When you insist that you *need* to get married, what you are really saying to God is this: *God, your power is insufficient. Your grace is insufficient. Your presence is insufficient. Your love for me is insufficient. Your help for me is insufficient. Your presence in my life is insufficient. God, You are insufficient!*

Satan zeros in and encourages this type of thinking. He will show you a parade of seemingly happily married couples. He will attempt to shroud you in a cloud of loneliness. He will place the army of potential suitors who are disastrously wrong for you in your path. Then, the next thing you know, you're wasting your life looking for somebody to make you whole. Satan encourages you to become a regular at happy hours, and at weddings where you don't even know the bride or groom. The world is filled with unhappy, unfulfilled couples. If you're single now, enjoy your singleness, learn all you can about yourself from it. Once you take this attitude, you will be amazed at the potential the Lord will place in your path. If you get married, bless the Lord! If you don't get married, bless the Lord!

Some of you may be missing out on the true blessings of life by waiting on some dream phantom person who, you are convinced, is out there somewhere. Forever pursuing the phantom is a trick of Satan. Let me suggest a way to turn the tables: consider the "dream" person to be you. Only if you become the person in your fantasy can you ever hope to attract that type of individual in the real world. Proof of your love and respect for the person you aim to become is the way you honor yourself. You refuse to cast your pearls to the swine, you refuse to compromise your morals and your principles.

You have decided to become Successfully Single.

When people participate in our Successfully Single workshop, it's as if a giant weight has been lifted from their shoulders. They discover they can be themselves instead of always trying to be somebody else in hopes of attracting the ideal mate they have in their minds. They give themselves permission to get on with their lives, without the burden of being, doing, and acting for someone else.

Singleness is a gift, a period when you can learn about yourself and use the process to become the best person you can become. Tami Johnson, a member of our congregation, learned this the hard way. She was, like too many of us, brought up to believe the myth of marriage. But then, one Sunday, she sat in the Windsor Village congregation during a sermon on relationships.

She listened to the definition of a God-blessed relationship and she immediately knew that absolutely *none* of its parameters were being met by her longtime, long-suffering relationship.

So she ended the relationship.

"I just told him that we weren't growing, weren't getting

closer, weren't meeting each other's needs," she says. "He would propose, but it didn't make sense. Because the relationship was clearly not at a point where anybody should be thinking about marriage."

Then, do you know what Ms. Johnson did? Somebody reading this book is thinking, "She went out and found somebody new!" Human nature occasionally encourages us to date someone "on the rebound," as the saying goes. Dating "on the rebound" occurs when you're hurt from a broken relationship and you date someone while the hurt is still stinging. You date in spite of not being ready. The God-blessed route is the route that Tami Johnson took. She learned to become Successfully Single before stepping back into the dating arena.

"I stopped dating," she says. "It's been over a year now. I get offers all the time. There's a person in Church who interests me and we often talk. But this time it's different. I'm getting to know him first as a person. It's not like I have to go out with him. If things develop, fine. If they don't, that's fine, too. The sense of panic and urgency has been lifted. I'm prepared to spend the rest of my life as a single person if I have to, and I believe the Bible supports that."

In the meantime, she's freed herself from the endless search, the knee-jerk mentality of "Could this be the one?" each time any man steps into her field of vision. She has regained an extraordinary amount of time in her life. Time to devote to her growth personally, spiritually, and professionally. "I no longer have the emotional baggage that comes from a bad relationship," she says. "My singleness has become a blessing."

By becoming Successfully Single, she's put herself in the position to be ready if God places the right person in her life. Blessedly, she has also properly positioned herself to be Successfully Single—period—whether she ever gets married or not!

How do you become Successfully Single?

1. *Realize that marriage is an option, not a commandment.* Yes, I am fully aware of God's exhortation to Adam and Eve: "Be fruitful and multiply." But marriage is not a necessary condition for being blessed, loved, or accepted by God. Don't subject yourself to undue pressure. In fact, as you read God's "Faith Hall of Fame" in Hebrews 12, singles are bountifully represented.

2. *Become yourself.* You read me right. Before you can become ready to truly know another, you must become—and remain—yourself. Become an individual, able to stand on your own two feet. The Jungian psychological term for this process is *individuation*. The simple layman's definition of *individuation* is a journey, which takes you from where you are to where you should be emotionally and relationally within yourself. The individuation process empowers you to break loose from your family origin issues, parental expectations, and peer pressure. To become individuated is to become yourself, find your own path, and be able to truly stand as an individual in the highest sense of the word.

You're not going to have to look very long at a person to determine whether he or she has embarked upon—much less completed—the process of individuation. This is one trait that is going to show, if you take time to look. And I mean to look honestly, without the blinders of physical attraction or mental denial. Codependency has become a modern plague because too many people look to another person for their affirmation—relationally, financially, and spiritually. Only when you allow God to create your life, and your own means of financial and spiritual support, can you truly be free.

If the person you're dating now is just like the person you were unsuccessfully dating two years ago, if your relationships seem to be a never-ending loop of woe, problems replicating themselves repeatedly, then it's likely that you're fishing for a mate with the wrong bait. Folks who do a lot of fishing will tell you: different kinds of fish require different kinds of bait. If you're fishing in the same funky pond you were fishing in three years ago, you're going to be pulling up the same fools you threw out last time you fished there. You need to change your bait, your attitude, your fishing location. If you do most of your fishing in nightclubs and you've thrown out everything you've caught, quit fishing in nightclubs. If you do most of your fishing in your gym and your catches have been unsuccessful, quit fishing in gyms. If you fish for a mate with anything but integrity, dignity, and truth, then you're deluding both your prospective mate and yourself.

Recently, a member of Windsor Village told me about how she had spent years fishing for a mate with lures of superficiality: first using her appearance, then using pretended innocence, and finally using seeming helplessness. In searching for someone who would simply love her, she meandered from one relationship to another, the failures mounting up over the years—relationships built on lies, deceit, and trickery. Finally, she realized her mistake: "I discovered that we are deceiving ourselves when we think we have to go fishing at all," she says. "As heirs to the throne, we should be content in whatever situation we're in. We should trust and love God with all of our heart. If we do that, everything else will fall into place. God knows every single thing about us, every character trait we have. Once we begin to rely on Him, to love Him completely, then we no longer miss having a mate and no longer feel compelled to go fishing. Then, one day, you'll discern and discover someone who loves you for who you are. God does not call you, nor has God created you, to 'go fishing.' God has called you to love yourself, others, and God."

THE DEVIL OF DOOMED RELATIONSHIPS

I met a woman who was in a longtime relationship with a man who was unwilling to communicate, compromise, or even listen to her.

"I was dating Satan and as long as I was dating Satan, he loved me," she told me. "But as soon as I quit him, he began riding my back."

I thought it was an incredibly revealing quote. True love, ultimately, is not controlling, not manipulative, and not conditional—three salient attributes of a Satan-induced relationship. Satan will typically ride your back if things are not going his way. As long as things are going his way—as long as you follow his directives—he "loves" you. If not, he'll give you, through the humans he's using, a true taste of hell. That's Satan's job.

Every Sunday, when I stand at that pulpit and talk about God-blessed relationships, I look at the faces of my congregation and just know I've hit a hundred nerves. Heads nod, eyes water, and folks sometimes squirm in their seats uncomfortably. The statistics on dysfunctional, destructive, and devil-driven relationships are shocking in America, where we have been severely lacking in even elementary lessons in How to Love.

I frequently offer my congregation a simple formula for determining if they're already involved in a God-blessed relationship. There are three simple parameters:

1. The relationship meets your needs.
2. The relationship is growing.
3. The relationship doesn't require your constantly asking God for forgiveness.

These three simple parameters have opened a big door in many a relationship among the members of my congregation. God-blessed relationships are very simple, very clean partnerships: the partners love each other, meet each other's needs, grow in their love, and act in accordance with God's will. Dysfunctional relationships, in contrast, are complicated messes. They tend to be dictatorships instead of partnerships, jumbles of Satanic stuff, peppered with arguments and constantly clouded in confusion. Once you can step outside of your emotions and look at your relationship analytically, you'll immediately know if it's God-blessed, or Satan-cursed.

One Sunday, a woman at Windsor Village listened to a relationship sermon, her husband at her side. Every word hit her like an arrow, she told me afterward, bursting the balloons of denial she had carried in her mind about her husband. She was forever catching him in lies. She couldn't trust him any more, much less love him, especially after she found the deposit slips in his lipstick-stained jacket for the secret bank accounts he'd opened in his name with the proceeds he was supposed to be depositing into their joint account from her business. She was making a respectable income, but her checks were bouncing regularly. She'd given him money to buy a car; she found out he'd leased the car and kept the cash for himself.

If you feel as if you can't trust him. If you catch him in incessant lies. If your relationship isn't growing. If you're always having to go to God for forgiveness. Then, obviously, an adjustment needs to be made and the issues need to be identified and addressed.

The message of the sermon was a summary of this woman's life. She was no different from a hundred other persons that day. You will find them in virtually every neighborhood, shopping center, health club, and corporate office: lying, cheating, deceptive men and women ever ready to vacuum you—mind, body, and soul—like a Hoover vacuum cleaner. Fools with all of the attributes of a dog except fidelity.

After Church, the woman described above tried to discuss the sermon with her mate.

"Did you hear today's message?" she asked him.

"Yeah," he grunted.

"What did you think about it?"

"I have no comment," he said.

He wouldn't listen, much less talk—another sign of a dysfunctional mate. Instead, he got in his car and left, taking his wife's money, the car, the business she had created, and every visible means of support. It would turn out to be a Godsend. Because if you're in a dysfunctional relationship, a relationship beyond healing and reconciliation, a relationship filled with deceit and lies, then you've got to get down to ground zero before you can begin to rebuild. You'll have to resist the urge to "fix" your mate, an urge that leads so many good-intentioned men and women into an endless cycle of wasted time.

COMMUNICATE

If you need wisdom—if you want to know what God wants you to do—ask Him, and He will gladly tell you. He will not resent your asking. But when you ask Him, be sure that you really expect Him to answer, for a doubtful mind is as unsettled as a wave of the sea that is driven and tossed by the wind.

—JAMES 1:5–6

How do you know when to begin, or end, a relationship with someone? First, you must truly know him or her. In Genesis, it is written of Adam and Eve, "They were naked before each other." This can be taken both literally and metaphorically. In order to enter a God-blessed relationship, you must stand psychologically naked before your partner; you must be willing to disrobe, to risk and empty yourself. You must be willing to let your prospective mate know your issues, secrets, and facts.

The key is, of course, communication.

Just as Adam and Eve knew little about each other, today's mates must learn to communicate before they can delve deeper in their love. One pivotal key to God-blessed relationships is commu-

nication. If you expect to be in a good and faithful and fruitful relationship with God, you must learn to communicate. If you expect
to have good, faithful, and fruitful relationships with your spouse,
mate, children, in-laws, coworkers, friends, or enemies, you must
communicate! Poor communication causes wars. Poor communication causes senseless murders, decimated marriages, and disinte-
grated business partnerships. Poor communication is the killer of
relational harmony. The word *communication* has as its root word
commune, which means "to have in common." When you are communicating with someone, then you have something in common.
You are exchanging ideas, thoughts, hurts, feelings. The other person understands what you are saying, and ideally the other person
even understands *why* you are saying what you are saying. Communication involves exchange, synergy, rhythm, flow.

The author/theologian John A. Sanford compares communication to playing ball. When you do or say something that the other
person does not understand and the ball of communication goes
over his or her head, then communication breaks down. I don't
care how well you said it, I don't care how many fancy words you
used, I don't care how long you prayed before you said it; if the
other person didn't catch the ball, you didn't communicate. Additionally, when you say to somebody, "You're no good! You're just
like your daddy!" you're playing hardball. Folks don't respond well
to hard balls. That is not communication; hardball communication
sparks disagreements, divorces, and wars.

Some folks believe that to communicate is to lecture. They're
wrong. Likewise, when you decide to change the rules, announce
that the rules are being changed. That messes up the whole ebb and
flow of the game when you change the rules. That softball doesn't
bounce like the basketball. So if I'm going to change the rules, I
need to announce, "I am now going to throw a softball." "It's no
longer one bounce and a catch, as was the case with the basketball.

Expect a direct throw with the softball." Give them some preparation. That's what communication is all about.

Communication involves two present parties, never a third party that's not present. Anytime you hear somebody talking about someone who's not present—anytime you hear some *"He said/she said/you said/they said"*—don't be a fool and take gossip as the Gospel. If you heard that someone said something bad about you, go to the source! Go to them lovingly and say, "I don't know if this is true or not, but let me tell you what I heard." Now, if they did say what you heard they said about you, that's another issue. You need to know that, too! But at least give the third party the opportunity to communicate.

Then, once they begin the communication process, let them speak! Don't interrupt. If you're a chronic *interrupter,* you have to learn how to let other folks talk. We've all been in a conversation with somebody who wants to complete our sentences. Satan does not want the communication to take place. He does not want a simple exchange to take place; he does not want the expressions of joy and pain to take place. He wants to step in and intercept what's going on. He wants unexpressed thoughts and feelings to remain in your head and gut so he can exacerbate and discombobulate, causing resentment, anger, and shame. Now, you need to be alert and prayerful and know when Satan is moving in and intercepting your communication patterns.

The pursuit of effective communication can be risky, however. One of the most common risks, which deters people from communicating, is conflict. Whenever two or more persons engage in communication, there will be conflict. But conflict, in and of itself, is not bad. In fact, conflict is an essential ingredient in all God-blessed relationships. When there is no conflict, someone in the relationship is not thinking, not talking, not listening or lying. When two normal people communicate, conflict will naturally occur. If you're in a relationship devoid of conflict, then you're most likely in an unhealthy, distant relationship. Two normal people are bound to disagree on something at some point. The goal is not to let your communication end with your conflict. Work through it, and you will progress to a new level of intimacy and communication. Manage conflict; don't allow conflict to manage you.

WHAT YOU MUST KNOW
BEFORE THE FIRST KISS

A member of my congregation and I recently began to discuss what questions a single person should ask someone they're thinking about getting to know better. I quickly assembled a list of critical criteria. As we looked at our list, an interesting thing happened. We learned that it's not merely a list of questions for you to ask your prospective date or spouse or partner—these are questions you must also ask yourself. Because, as we've discussed, if you don't know yourself first, then how can you be ready to truly know somebody else?

Here is the list of critical questions to ask others and to know about yourself:

"What—or whom—do you worship?" Human beings are inherently worshiping creatures. We all worship somebody or something. In his book *Shattering the Gods Within,* David Allen highlights the point that we become the object of our worship. Which is to say, what you worship is what you eventually become. If you worship money, you become more materialistic. If you worship power, you become power-hungry. It is critical to understand who or what you or the person with whom you're considering a relationship worships. I've discovered that you can tell what someone worships by looking at their calendar and checkbook. How is your time spent? How is your money spent? Pay special attention. For your time and your money, follow your heart. Is the person with whom

you're jumping into bed worshiping her money, cars, jewelry, and wine cellar before God? You need to know. Is he worshiping himself? Self-worshipers can be particularly pernicious, because they are apt to view themselves as "mini-gods," deserving inordinate doses of praise and adoration. Some folks call these individuals egomaniacs or narcissists.

Who you allow into the inner concentric circles of your life is going to have a dramatic effect on who you are and what you become.

"What kind of relationship do you have with your mother and/or father?" Be concerned about how a person communicates with his or her own mother or father, because if they would 'dis' their mama or daddy, what do you think they're gonna do to you? Their parents clothed them, fed them, watered them, and they still 'dissed' them? What makes you think they won't 'dis' you?

Pay special attention to your current or prospective mate's "leave-and-cleave" quotient. As the Bible implies, a man shall leave his mama, daddy, girlfriends, golf clubs, tennis racket, and pool sticks and be joined to his wife. Likewise, a woman will leave her mother, father, sister, brother, dolls, boyfriends, and girlhood home and all the interfamilial rites and secrets contained therein. And the two shall become one flesh. Nothing or nobody should be closer to you than God and your spouse.

"What makes you cry? What makes you laugh? What are your dreams?" Show me the person who cannot cry and I will show you someone out of touch with his or her emotions. Jesus wept. Jesus was the most powerful man who ever walked the earth, but He wept. God made tears to be shed. God didn't create any part of us to be wasted. If you're learning how to cry, that's a different matter. Ask yourself, "What brings me pain?" "What brings me joy?" If you're considering developing a relationship with someone who can't laugh, can't cry with passion, do not fall into the trap of thinking that once you

marry or contractually bond with them that their tears and passion will burst forth like water through a dam. If they are not crying and filled with passion now, they certainly won't be after you say "I do."

After you determine what, if anything, makes them cry, ask them about their dreams. "What do you envision as God's preferred future for your life?" "What does God have in store for you?" If you can both ask and answer that question, you are one step ahead of Satan himself. Do not enter any significant relationship with anybody without knowing the motivations of their laughter, tears, and dreams.

"How many children have you fathered or mothered? Where are the children? Who has the custody? How much time do you spend with them?" As someone who provides marital counseling for thousands of people, I'm forever amazed at some of the information people do not have and do not know about their prospective mates. Think of yourselves as a detective, forever trying to prevent the crime that can cost you your life.

"Have you been married? How many times? How long ago? What happened?" Let's say that you've been married three times, and the breakup was always the other person's fault. You might think this is a positive since it was always the other person who was at fault, not you. Where is your accountability? You're choosing the wrong folk. There's something faulty with your pickin' process. You must examine yourself before you proceed in this relationship.

"If you were to receive a million dollars today, what would you do with it?" This question is gauged to tell you a whole lot about a man or woman. You ask some folk what they would do with a cool million and some of them would say, "I'd buy a Jaguar." Or "I would pay off my Christmas bills." That speaks volumes right there. These folks are car-conscious and Christmas-conscious. It is real important to understand your prospective mate's relationship with money, long before you jump into a relationship with them. The answer to this question will give you an indication as to whether

you're talking to an investor or a consumer, a saver or a spender, a financial winner or loser. Why are they the way they are? And what, if anything, are they willing to change? Address this issue before going too far. Avoid being manipulated, snarled, or wooed by someone's money.

"What experience in your life has brought you the greatest joy? The greatest sorrow? And most important, how have you processed it?" I meet with a group of men each month in a Bible-study group. Recently, we've been discussing how unprocessed pain *inside* us becomes anger *outside* of us. Into every person's life a little pain will fall. The question is whether you will process your anger in a healthy way. The annals of failure and disgrace are filled with folks who had everything going for them but didn't know how to process change. They couldn't handle success or failure successfully. They couldn't handle their blessing blessedly. Their inability to process their pain literally pulled them down. You need to learn how to express and process your pain—and how your prospective partner processes theirs! The inability or even unwillingness to express joy or sorrow speaks to the essence of one's emotional quotient.

"What is your three-, five-, ten-year vision for your life spiritually, financially, relationally?" Individuals who can't see their future usually haven't taken the time to search for it. Do you want to attach yourself to someone who floats through life like a feather on the wind? It doesn't take a crystal ball to have a vision for your future; find out what your prospective mate envisions for him or herself. As it is written in Proverbs, "Without a vision, people perish." Likewise, without people, a vision can perish. What is God's vision for your life?

"What are your addictions?" Let me offer my personal testimony regarding this point. Over two years ago, my wife, Suzette, said to me, "I believe you are a workaholic." At the time, she might have been right—although it really "teed me off" initially. The truth is

not afraid of inquiry. The truth is not afraid of questions; it is only when folks hook us where we live that we get sensitive and defensive. If you have an addiction, you have conditions; understand them and you'll know what drives them. Realize and address your addictions. Denial can kill you.

"When you die, what do you expect your friends—and enemies—to say about you? What do you want God to say about you?" If you want your friends to say you are honorable and trustworthy, and you have not started living a life of honor and trustworthiness, why not? Practice makes perfect. You have got to have a commercial before the program. Ask your prospective mate or partner to compose a eulogy for him or herself. Then, listen carefully. It will be an illuminating peek into their hearts—and minds. But first, compose your own eulogy. Pour your emotions into it; let it represent all you hope to become. Then, once you know what you want, walk with God toward creating your ultimate vision of yourself. You will have achieved one of the greatest gifts you can give yourself and God: self-knowledge. And then, and only then, can you be prepared for the glory of a God-blessed relationship.

THE EIGHT CHARACTERISTICS OF
MR./MS. RIGHT

Okay, so now you think you've found Mr. or Ms. Right. Everything about them seems presentable. But you know by now that God-blessed relationships are not happenstance, close encounters, or psychological quickies. God-blessed, lasting relationships take time, thought, and work. How do you know if Mr. or Mrs. Right is what he or she seems to be? At Windsor Village, we've devised sort of a relationship checklist comprising of eight required characteristics to look for in a spouse or mate. Let me share that list with you.

1. Ensure that your spouse/mate is someone with whom you can be "Equally Yoked."

As it is written in 2 Corinthians 6:14: *"Do not be unequally yoked together with unbelievers. For what fellowship has righteousness with lawlessness? And what communion has light with darkness?"* Simply put, the verse is advising against becoming "unequally yoked," whether it is imbalance of belief, expectations, philosophy, trust, work, or love. God-blessed relationships should be as balanced as a scale. This may seem fundamental, but the world is filled with unequally yoked couples. If you are unequally yoked, you'll be going one way while your spouse/mate will be going the other. You're in the Church and he or she is out of the Church; you'll love the Lord, they won't love the Lord; you want to come to Church/school/work; they won't want to go to Church/school/work. You'll have a problem on your hands; they won't be able to see it. An unequally yoked spouse/mate is forever presenting real, fundamental conflicts in your everyday agenda. God-blessed relationships are journeys of growth and fulfillment. You can't make that journey if your partner is always pulling you in the opposite direction.

2. Look beyond the wrapper.

I hear it all the time, the attributes of the exterior: *"But he or she makes $75,000 a year! But he's so fine! But she's got all these frequent-flyer miles and all I have to do is pack my tennis racket and pack my golf clubs and I'm gone!"* While you are looking at *what* he or she *has*, focus on *who* he or she *is*. Satan's biggest trick is to lure you into a self-defeating relationship with the eye candy of money, beauty, and fame.

3. Make sure the person you're spending time with is single.

Again, this is elementary. But I see untold numbers of married folks dating persons other than—or in addition to—their spouses. You think you've been to Heartbreak Hotel. You start dating somebody who promises, *"I'm getting divorced, it's just a matter of time,"* and you could be checking in for an extended stay. These people will invariably start telling you about everything their spouses are not doing for them and everything that you do for them, giving you a nonstop rundown on their no-good, low-down, silly wife or sorry husband. You get your hopes, dreams, and desires all built up, only to have him or her turn his or her behind on you and go back to his or her spouse, and then you are destroyed. Several members of my congregation have told me, "I *prefer* a married person." Most who prefer a relationship with a married person do so because they want someone who places a premium on low or no commitment. If you're thinking like this, there is something in your background, in your psyche, that causes you to pursue a relationship disaster. You need to know what it is, then do some serious work upon your problem.

4. *Make certain the person you're spending time with is sober.*

Make sure they're not drunk on booze, drugs, or most of all, themselves. Now, if you're dating someone or you're married to someone who has a history of alcohol, substance, or ego abuse, and they're working through it, that's beautiful. I'm not talking about that. I'm talking about these folk who are still drunk and in denial. Those are the folks who will attach themselves to you with suckers. Pretty soon, you'll find yourself asking questions like "Baby, have you seen my ring? my watch? the car?" And finally, "Baby, have you seen my life?" If you figure once you married them it would be all right, you are wrong. God-blessed relationships don't involve "babysitting" adults. If you find yourself babysitting your spouse/mate, it is time to seek help, or in some cases, get out.

5. *Make sure your potential spouse/mate is sane.*

In other words, you're dating somebody and they have a history of calling folks' houses and hanging up, or going over to somebody's house in their car and sitting in the car down the corner waiting to see who drives up. Would you buy a new car on passion alone? No. You would have an inspection and look under the hood. Do the same with your prospective spouse/mate.

6. *Make sure your potential spouse/mate has some spunk.*

In the Old Testament, it was firmly understood that a person who had a sense of humor had a close walk with God. Make sure your prospective spouse/mate has a sense of humor, a little glee about himself or herself. A too tightly wound spring will break. When someone is so tightly wound up that they can't laugh at themselves, consider it a warning sign! My mother used to tell me, "A person's sense of humor will take a relationship, especially a marriage, a long way." If you don't have a sense of humor, get one! Really. Cultivate spirit and lightness in your life. Merriment is medicine for the soul. Proverbs 17:22 reminds us that a merry heart does good, like medicine.

7. *Make sure they have a healthy relationship with money.*

I can't stress this point too much. If you're dating somebody who never leaves a tip or pays for a meal, you're dating somebody you need to leave. If they're unemployed and looking for a job, that's different. But if they're employed and act like a nickel is as heavy as a manhole cover, consider it a red flag! Pay special attention to how your prospective spouse/mate handles money. If he or she is a scrooge or a spendthrift, you don't want to wait until after the wedding to discover why. Do they drive a car that's bigger than the apartment they live in? Do they consistently spend more money than they earn on luxury items? Do they have clothes in the closet with the sales tags still on them? Remember, the devil uses the issue of money to cause many an argument. You need to have some working understanding as to where the other person is on the stewardship issue.

8. *Make sure the person has some sense of security and self-esteem.*

These two things—security and self-esteem—go hand in hand. Some people tend to define themselves in relation to their significant others. If they don't have enough sense of self to stand successfully on their own, they'll never make successful mates. Discover a person's issues before walking down that aisle. If you do not know joy right now, do not expect marriage or a mate to introduce you to joy. In other words, if you're miserable and single, and you think getting married is going to resolve your misery, then you're apt to be miserable *and* married.

WHAT GOOD BUSINESS AND GOOD MARITAL RELATIONSHIPS SHARE

In the May 25, 1998, issue of *Fortune* magazine, Ram Charan, a corporate adviser to Fortune 500 companies, offers "five broad steps" that CEOs of newly merged large companies could follow in order to create a synergistic "social and operational architecture to make a two-headed operation come together."

Ram's five steps are:

1. Agree on a definition of success;
2. Acknowledge each other's strengths and define roles accordingly;
3. Make communication a priority;
4. Build trust; and
5. Get to know the other guy's people.

I found it interesting that Charan's principles could also apply to married couples. Let's examine these steps one by one. I suggest that you pull out pen and paper and that you and your spouse give your thoughts on these five points in writing independently of each other. Then, sit down and compare notes. Once your two perspectives have been honestly and thoroughly examined on paper, develop strategies for reconciling the two statements into one. If you and your spouse, or fiancé, reach an impasse or significant "bone of contention," then please seek the direction of a competent, effective third-party counselor.

Here are the points to consider:

1. *Agree on a definition of success.* Determine how you and your spouse define a successful marriage. What does it look like? What are some necessary steps that must be taken in order to achieve this success? You and your spouse, or fiancé, need to develop a working understanding of a successful marriage. After all, how can a couple expect to move in the same direction if they do not know what their goals are, much less agree on a common goal?

2. *Acknowledge each other's strengths and define roles accordingly.* Marriage requires teamwork. Each member of any effective team understands his or her role in the team. A good leader is able to position and play the team members according to their strengths so that the members' collective efforts are maximized. Married people can ill afford to be jealous of their spouse's strengths. These demons must be addressed and cast out immediately! Your spouse should bring out the best in you, not inspire envy, jealousy, or a competitive spirit. It's "We win" or "We lose." Not "I win" or "You lose." Learn to identify, acknowledge, deploy, and celebrate your spouse's strengths. Then, allow and encourage your spouse to use these strengths to take your marriage to the next level. Who does what in the household should be a function of who does what best. In my house, Suzette handles the day-to-day financial operations. Tell your EGO—which can be thought of as Edging God Out—to sit down. Allow your best combination of strengths to bless your marriage. Spouses should bring out the best in each other, inspiring excellence, joy and wholeness.

3. *Make communication a priority.* Talk, talk, talk and listen, listen, listen. We've already learned how to listen earlier in this chapter; this is a reit-

eration of its importance. If you want to offer the devil a head start on your marriage, then don't make communication a priority. When your spouse asks you how you feel, tell her! The devil thrives on miscommunication. Remember his first move in the Garden of Eden? He lied to Eve, lied on God, and lied around Adam. He's still lying and miscommunicating today. When the devil tells you that a significant marital issue will go away, so there's no need to discuss it with your spouse, he's lying! The Bible reminds us that the devil is a liar and the truth his not in him. The busiest and most complicated agendas should be rearranged and cleared to make room for communication. Poor or no communication will set your marriage up for a one-day ticket from hell.

4. *Build trust.* In his *Fortune* article, Ram Charan writes, "Growth, the whole point of these new mergers, can be critically stunted if the partners are competing with each other or if they are so deferential that one will never presume to speak for the other." Spouses should grow in their marriages, and trust is the water that creates growth. How do you make trust grow? You show your spouse that you trust him in very real ways. Your marriage, which is supposed to grow, cannot develop if mistrust prevails. If pre-existing issues have caused walls to be erected, then those issues need to be addressed and reconciled. Ask your spouse, *What do I need to do for you to establish trust in me?*

5. *Get to know the other guy's people.* Ah! How many times have you heard a bride or groom say, "I'm not marrying the parents or siblings." That's true, but you'd best know who these parents or siblings are. If your spouse's folks, or "people," are fools, you need to know. Although there are always exceptions, I've discovered that the adage "The fruit doesn't fall too far from the tree" is usually true. If the parents are "a case," then beware. I always encourage engaged couples to attend each other's family gatherings or reunions. This can be informative. When you attend your future spouse's family function for the first or second time, your goal is to learn, not teach. Listen, don't talk too much. Follow, don't lead. Family reunions can be extremely rewarding and enlightening events. If you're smart, you'll be able to

learn the reasons behind your mate's actions. You'll understand why some values are more important to him or her than others. You're apt to also learn some crucial personal history. Never forget: knowledge is power! Get to know your spouse's folks! But go to in-law-to-be or in-law-family events as a humble student, not a haughty teacher, as an astute observer, not an obstructionist. If you cannot go in this spirit, then take it as a sign that you are not ready to take advantage of this potentially tremendous opportunity. I'm not advising against establishing boundaries to prevent your in-laws from invading, and abusing, your personal space. I'm merely saying take time to know them. Remember: loving somebody is one thing; knowing *how* to love them is related but undeniably different. The truth is not afraid of inquiry.

To help you get started on your journey of God-blessed marital relationships, allow me to offer seven areas to which Ram Charan's five broad steps can be applied. These seven areas represent aspects of a marriage or engagement that are explicitly addressed or implicitly operative in most God-blessed marital relationships. Although this list is not exhaustive, it certainly contains areas necessary for establishing a solid foundation.

The areas are:

1. Faith
2. Future
3. Family
4. Friends
5. Finances
6. Fun
7. Feelings

What are your relationship's strengths and weaknesses in each of these seven areas? Most troubles in marriages and can be traced to one, some, or all of these areas.

Conflict, as we will discuss further in the next section, is a sign of growth. When marriages are growing, conflict is both normal and healthy. Unresolved, recurring conflicts between spouses, on the other hand, can be downright ugly and cause a lot of pain. When these types of conflicts occur frequently and you are able to resolve them in a healthy manner, then that's an "opportunity" to grow both individually and as a couple. When these conflicts occur frequently, but you are not able to resolve them, then that's an impasse. Impasses can be marriage breakers, so I suggest that you immediately seek competent counsel to help resolve it.

When conflicts occur infrequently and you are able to resolve them yourself, then "it came to pass." It's just another day in the life of a marriage. When conflicts occur infrequently but you are not able to resolve them in a healthy manner, then that is an "issue." Issues can become marriage breakers if left to their own evolution. I encourage you not to allow multiple issues to accumulate. Sit down and make them go away. See the chart below:

		Can Be Resolved by the Spouses Themselves	
		Yes	No
Frequently	No	It came to pass	An issue
encountered in your marriage	Yes	An opportunity	An impasse

USING CONFLICT AS A KEY

As Ichak Adizes states in his book *Corporate Lifecycles,* "to live means to continuously solve problems. The fuller a life is, the more complex the problems are that must be resolved." In order to be a good and faithful steward of your life, you must be able to continuously solve problems. We have been taught to associate trouble or problems with negativity. A person is without problems only when there is no change. When there is no change, there is no growth. When there is no growth, you are near death. Change and conflict are signs of life. If you have problems due to change and growth, then congratulations!

Folks with big Faith can handle big problems! Conflict is one way God uses to develop and grow your relationship. No risks, no reward. No investment, no return. No cross, no crown. No conflict, no growth! Satan tends to score his points in the conflict arena when couples struggle with how their conflict will be processed. Do you manage conflict or does conflict manage you? Adults who grew up in homes where conflicts were poorly managed tend to shy away from conflict altogether—and understandably so. Poorly managed conflict almost always causes pain and confusion—and that, of course, is Satan's breeding ground.

Additionally, some adults shy away from conflict because they grew up in homes where there was very little, if any, outward manifestation of conflict. These folks, without the benefit of enlightenment, tend to think that any manifestation of conflict is a sign of irreversible doom. But conflict is both healthy and desirable. Short-term conflict creates long-term power in relationships.

It is tempting for some of us to fall victim to the Karl Marx Conflictless Syndrome, described in the book *Corporate Lifecycles*. It seems that Marx tried to negate conflict as though it were a pathological development. Some marriage partners do the same thing: they sweep issues under the rug by ignoring spousal habits that are detrimental not only to the relationship but to the spouses themselves. They internalize their pain, guilt, or shame. They withhold information that could deepen their relationship. Doing this is an invitation to the devil; your molehills will eventually become mountains that you will certainly have to deal with. Then conflict becomes not a tool for growth but a battleground for war.

There are rules to disagree by, however. I've learned a very effective system to communicate in conflict from the Houston psy-chotherapist Michael Thomas, who presented the following illu-minating information about communication to our Church. According to the founder of transactional analysis, Eric Berne, hu-mans, if older than two, pretty much communicate from one of three basic ego states: the parent, the adult, and the child.

Each state has the following attributes:

The parent ego state can be either critical or nurturing.

The adult ego state is rational, even in anger.

The child ego state can be compliant, as in the Goodie Two-Shoes type, or the rebellious child, as in the acting-out type of child.

Michael Thomas showed our Confirmation Class group how people in couples communicate with each other from these different ego states when it comes to conflict. He gave the following example: A wife is confronting her spouse about not doing what he said he was going to do—in this case, neglecting to pick up the laundry.

She has three choices in confronting her mate:

First, she can confront as a critical, accusatory parent: pointing the finger, being condescending, controlling, authoritative: *"This is the third time this week you promised you were going to do something and you didn't do it!"*

Second, she can confront him from the child's perspective: She can pick up the clothes from the laundry herself and pout about it.

Finally, she could confront him from the healthiest perspec-tive, the adult: *"Listen, we've got to talk. I'm not sure what's going on. I'm working this extra job because we need money. I'm concerned about this. What's the best way for us to work together to resolve this situation?"*

Just as the woman could respond from one of three different positions, her counterpart could also respond three different ways:

If she comes in and uses the critical, accusatory parent ego—which, Michael Thomas says, is generally how it happens in relationships—he will probably feel threatened, become defensive, and counter her argument. He'll come from a parent perspective of his own, matching her criticism and accusations with some of his. When parent meets parent, power meets power. You have no winners from that position, you simply have a standoff.

Second, if she comes from the parent perspective, he could react from the child's: making excuses. The more he makes excuses and comes from the child, the more he reinforces her coming from the parent. He gives her permission to come from the parent, leading them into a never-ending cycle.

The third way, however, is the healthiest way, the God-blessed route: If the woman comes in ranting and raving, again coming from the parent, the man can come from the adult perspective. He can say, *"Whoa, time out. Look at how you're talking to me. You're treating me like a child. Let's see how we can achieve our common goals here."*

For the most part, it's healthiest to come from the adult perspective in any argument, whether you find yourself the accuser of the accused. What's critical to recognize is that you're coming from it when you're coming from it. Remember, Satan destroys relationships by interfering with, and interrupting, communication patterns. Satan will tempt you to come from the child and accusing-parent positions, pitting you as persecutor versus victim. He strives to keep people from coming from adult perspective, which is, of course, the only healthy way to deal with conflict.

When you do something wrong, admit it, seek forgiveness. If you are unsure how, here's a list that might come in handy.

SIXTEEN WAYS TO WHUP THE DEMONS
IN YOUR MARRIAGE

1. For the times I failed to communicate my own feelings, forgive me.

2. For the times you hurt me and I did not tell you, forgive me.

3. For the times I listened with my mouth and then spoke with my ears, forgive me.

4. For the times I fussed when I should have felt, forgive me.

5. For the times I blamed you because it was less painful than facing myself, forgive me.

6. For the times I allowed my unprocessed inner pain to become outer anger, forgive me.

7. For the times I held you responsible for not meeting my unexpressed expectations, forgive me.

8. For all of the family secrets that affect me that I have not told you about, forgive me.

9. For the Divine difference(s) that you have made in my life and that I never told you about, forgive me.

10. For the times you were right and I was wrong and I never told you, forgive me.

11. For the times I told my family or friends more about me than I told you, forgive me.

12. For the times I told my family or friends more about my feelings about you than I told you, forgive me.

13. For my personal demons which I refuse to deal with, which affect me and subsequently you, forgive me.

14 For the times I used the children to get back at you, forgive me.

15. For the times I withheld lovemaking because I was on strike, forgive me.

16. For sharing "spousal love" with anybody other than you, forgive me.

Relationship Maintenance

*A friend never gets in your way unless you
happen to be going down.*

—Arnold Glasow

Let's now focus specifically on how to improve communication between spouses and mates. I've identified nine different ways that men can communicate deeply with their mates and nine ways that women can communicate with theirs. Some have been adapted from John Gray's book *Men Are from Mars, Women Are from Venus.* The first nine ways are from men to women. The second nine ways are from women to men.

Tell her you love her every day . . . every day! Remember the Stevie Wonder song, "I Just Called to Say I Love You"? That song contains an important kernel of advice. *Love shows signs!* If you never tell your woman you love her, then how is she going to know? Now, I'm not talking about empty words of love. If you don't mean it, don't say it. If somebody says they love you but they don't meet your needs or bring you joy, if you feel worse when you leave them than you did when you said hello, then no amount of empty exultations is going to help you. I don't care how fine she is; you can be 36–22–36 and be hell on wheels. You can be cut like Mr. Universe and be the devil's gift to womankind. But if you're in a committed relationship, it's critical that you tell your mate that you love her . . . every day!

Hug her daily. How do dogs, babies, children, and spouses become mean and angry? It's safe to say one aspect is the absence of physical contact from others. It's been said that we need four hugs a day for survival, eight hugs a day for maintenance, and twelve hugs a day for growth. My wife, Suzette, and I have gotten to the point where we know when we need a hug! It's one of the high points of our day. Sometimes, we just hug every day for preventive purposes. Sometimes, she'll look at me and say, "Baby, you need a hug." If you want to build communication and intimacy with your mate, *hug her every day!* Of course, some folks at some times are downright *unhuggable*. But, right at the nadir of her unhuggable-ness, that's when you need to give her the biggest hug that you can!

Practice Listening and ask specific questions about her day, while paying *attention*. This is the most difficult thing for many men. Men generally tend to be linear in their thinking. They're more bottom-line-oriented. They're apt to say, "What's up with this?" and "Let's make a decision . . . right now!" They're trained to push for results, outcomes, conclusions, whereas women require process. Women usually have a need to discuss, analyze, study options, determine feasibility and probability. Men must understand that this analytical aspect is not a negative. One of the reasons that God made both man and woman is that they're complementary. Men must under-stand that when women show their feelings, it doesn't mean they're fussing—they're just showing their feelings. I believe this is one reason why women outlive men: they have the ability to vent. Men tend to keep everything inside. Take the time to listen to your woman, without trying to fix, solve, or rationalize. Just listen. It's the best investment you can make in your relationship.

Typically, a woman is more apt to tell you how she feels, if asked. A man, on the other hand, when asked how he feels, is prone to tell you what he *thinks*. Men must learn to listen and ex-press their feelings based upon the needs of the relationship, not natural male proclivities.

Validate her feelings when she's upset. Even if you disagree with why she's upset, don't fall into the knee-jerk reaction that she doesn't have the right to be angry. Validate her feelings, then take time to understand why she is feeling a particular way. Nobody wants to be dissed. You're dissing your wife, mate, sister, or mother when you dispute her God-given right to *feel*. What she's feeling might not be appropriate to you at that moment, but her feelings are her own! She has a right to feel however she wants to feel at any given moment; if you don't understand this basic fact you are opening the door to misery.

Do not flick the television remote control. Every time I mention this one, a roar goes up in my congregation. Every man on the planet seems to have a natural inclination to change channels in the middle of whatever show his wife or mate is watching. Many women have to resort to actually hiding the remote control from their channel-changing mates. Put down that remote control! Do it now! Changing that channel is a signal that you are not even aware, much less concerned, about what your spouse is doing.

Show affection! Men are motivated by sight, women are motivated by touch. Men place value upon what they own; women place value on who they are and with whom they spend their lives. Traditionally, women are the caregivers in the home. To create a flourishing sense of communication, men must learn to do what women already instinctively know: show affection.

Have a date night, preferably without the children. Once you have established a date night, keep it. My wife and I have made our date night Friday night. I make it a priority. People know not to ask me to do anything on Friday night unless it's a life-or-death situation. Suzette has never accepted an engagement on Friday night without asking me first; I've never accepted one without asking her. If appointments for golf, handball, basketball, teatime, or the beauty shop are important enough to set and keep, then spending time with your spouse should be just as important, if not more important. If you're thinking, "I don't feel like dating my spouse again," consider it a sign that you *really* need a date night. I'm not talking about an expensive date. You can go to a $3 movie or simply out to get a 75-cent cup of coffee. You can simply sit home and watch a little TV and pop some popcorn. It's not *what* you do that's important; it's that you're doing it.

Give her a kiss and say goodbye before leaving. This sounds elementary. But with some folks, you know they're gone only because you heard the car start up and the door slam. Departure salutations are a sign of respect. It tells your spouse that she's important enough for you to say goodbye to her and kiss her before you go.

Show appropriate affection in public. If you walk five steps ahead of your spouse or mate, you're walking way too fast. Holding hands, an occasional hug, and maintaining some sense of eye and brain contact are essential. People have a need to be affirmed not only in private but in public. This sends a message to the world: "This person completes me."

Now that we've learned what men must do for their wives or mates, here are my own impressions of what women should do for their husbands or mates.

Tell him you honor him, at least daily! The Bible says "Husbands, love your wives." The Bible also says, "Wives, *honor* your husbands." I find it interesting that love would be given to the women, honor to the men. But it fits. Because just as most women have an inherent need for love, most men have a deep desire to feel honored, especially at home. The adage "A man's home is his castle" perfectly describes the way most men feel about their homes. It's a natural tendency. A woman might be running his world—as many women do—but a man has a basic need to feel as if he's worthy of honor. He might be unemployed, he may not have made a contribution toward the mortgage payment since the Mississippi was a creek, but within that man is a spark that can grow, especially if a woman takes time to feed him with honor. Wise women under-

238 THE GOSPEL OF GOOD SUCCESS

stand this basic male need. Wise women understand that you can catch more flies with honey than you can with vinegar! Even if he's not deserving of honor now, honor him for what you believe he can accomplish in the future. Say to yourself, "I am honoring him now, not for who he is today but for what he has the capacity to become tomorrow." Have Faith in him, pray for him, and give him the greatest gift: honor. The transformation can and will occur.

Hug him daily. Men have the same need for hugs that women do! Remember the formula: four hugs a day for survival, eight for maintenance, twelve for growth. He may be as grouchy as a junk-yard dog, but beneath the bluster is a little boy. Show him some affection. Give him a hug. And watch him melt before your eyes.

Do not compare him to other men, especially your daddy! How many times have you heard a woman say, "All men are dogs"? But all men, like all women, are individuals. I've never met a man who enjoys being compared with previous boyfriends, husbands, and especially, fathers. That said, let me offer a key to understanding your man. Some women tend to marry the mirror image of their father, just as some men tend to marry the mirror image of their mother. Sisters, if you have issues with your father, past or present, that are unresolved, consider the possibility that the same issues could be having a negative impact on your marriage. Some of the anger that *wives have toward their husbands* is precipitated or generated by residual anger they have toward their father. There are many scriptural examples of this. Your father may be deceased, so there's no way you can physically go back and make amends with him. But don't allow those issues to affect your relationship with your husband or mate. That's what grace and mercy and forgiveness are all about. Satan wants guilt and shame to be heaped on your marriage or partnership; he wants you shouldered and burdened with leftover pain and unresolved issues. Remember: your husband or mate is not your father. Cut the cord between the two in your mind.

Show appreciation for his income. You might think he needs to bring home more bacon. But honor what he is bringing home right now. If he's not bringing home anything, if he's sucking you down with dependency, that's another thing. But if the man is working, if he's doing his best to bring home a paycheck, then the best thing you can do is to honor what he is bringing home. As we've said, earning motivates men. Some men have even been tricked by Satan to believe that they are what they earn. Show him that he is more than a paycheck and watch that paycheck grow.

Do not belittle him in public. If you have an ax to grind, grind it at home. Public ax grinding is apt to remind your man of when his mother or some other adult female figure chastised him as a child. You want to remind him that you are his honey, not his mommy. You want to propel him into the future, not pull him back into the past. Understand that words can hurt. Don't belittle him in public, or in front of your children.

Look attractive. I believe women are motivated by touch, men are motivated by sight. Many a woman's style of dress drops off precipitously once she says "I do." I'm not talking about weight gain or loss, plastic surgery or liposuction. I'm talking about using what God gave you to look your absolute best. I've seen folks weigh 300 pounds and be well groomed. Brush your teeth, use mouthwash, comb your hair! *Spruce yourself up.* When you dress up and look better when you're going out with the girls than when you go out with your husband, you've got a demon swirling around your marriage.

Don't nag. Say it once, and if he doesn't get it, write him a note. I hear it all the time: "My wife/girlfriend/date says the same thing over and over again—and the way she said it last time is the same way she said it the first time." This makes a man insecure, makes him feel that you don't trust him enough to tell him once, that you feel you have to repeat everything to him as if he were a child in order for it to sink through his thick skull. Say it once and see if he acts upon it. If nothing is done, of course, then say it again. But don't get into the habit of repeating everything a dozen times.

Be patient with him while he is growing spiritually. Transformations take time. They're usually described as flashes of brilliant light, instantaneous realizations, immediate epiphanies. But more often than not, spiritual growth is a process that may take years to achieve. Be patient with your spouse or mate as he grows in his Faith in the Lord. Realize that merely the willingness to grow, to listen, to learn, is major step enough. Support him with patience and encouragement.

Show interest in his hobbies and support for his business decisions. That's important. A man views his business as an extension of himself. *Even if it doesn't work out, don't play him like a bass guitar.* He *knows* it didn't work out. Give him the space to not let it work out! Let him learn from his mistakes and press forward. Don't kick him for mistakes he's made in the past and mistakes you think he's about to make in the future.

GOD'S HIGHEST BLESSING

Carmen, the nationally known Christian singer-songwriter, once told me, "Your spouse is God's opinion of you." The thought references the spouse as a "reward" for what you have done or an indicator of what you're capable of doing. Since your spouse is your helpmate, your life is maximized when you're coupled with the person God wants you to have. Carmen's quote assumes, of course, that God has someone for each person who desires marriage and that everyone finds this person. Accordingly, then, a first-class spouse would imply that God perceives you as a first-class person, someone who has perhaps crawled through the valley of deception and now stands at the summit of God-blessed love.

Epilogue:
Becoming Whole

We are all born whole, and let us hope, will die whole. But somewhere early on our way, we eat one of the wonderful fruits of the tree of knowledge, things separate into good and evil, and we begin the shadow-making process; we divide our lives.

—ROBERT A. JOHNSON

IN THE BOOK OF JOHN, CHAPTER 5, JESUS ENCOUNTERS A man who has been ill for thirty-eight years. The man awaits healing with a great multitude—folks who are blind, lame, withered, or otherwise infirm—beside a pool in Bethesda, where, he had been advised, healing powers would arrive when bubbles appeared in the pool. While the broken man was waiting for the water to magically "bubble up," Jesus, having known the man had been ill a long time, asked him a pivotal question: *"Do you want to be made whole?"*

A simple, yet terribly significant inquiry! But instead of accepting Jesus' grace, instead of simply replying, "Yes," the man begins speaking out of a victim's mentality, blaming other people, systems, and processes. The sick man began playing the blame game, questioning his deliverance, instead of simply accepting it from the Master Healer.

Do you want to be made whole? Simply say, "Yes!" Then, begin to develop the belief system and behavior pattern that reflect your declaration. First you must *want* to become whole. It's so incredibly simple, yet so many of us make it so difficult. In order to re-

ceive, walk in, and live out our wholeness, we must want to be
whole!

The following seven-point self-inventory may be in order at
this point as you prepare your pathway to wholeness.

- Have you given yourself permission to be whole?
- Are you ready to receive the benefits and blessings which derive
  from becoming whole? Are you prepared to be a faithful steward of
  those benefits and blessings?
- Are you willing to pay the price to obtain and maintain your
  wholeness?
- Are you willing to lose broken friends who may become
  uncontrollably envious of your new wholeness?
- Are you willing to invest the virtues of self-control, self-discipline
  and focus in order to pursue your wholeness?
- When evil attacks you for becoming whole, will you be ready to
  fight to keep your wholeness?
- As you grow in wholeness, will you know how to defeat the demons
  of guilt, mediocrity, and insecurity and other demons which may,
  depending upon your family origin issues—and your moral,
  environmental, and social norms—cause you to implode while
  journeying on your path to wholeness?

IDENTIFY YOUR NEEDS

Before you can truly realize that the diverse pieces of your life were
Divinely designed to operate as a cohesive whole, you have to
know what these pieces are. The best way to do this is by identifying your needs. Everybody has needs—spiritual, financial, emotional, social, educational, and medical. Identifying your needs and
finding healthy ways to get your needs met are absolutely essential
to becoming whole.

The accompanying chart, entitled "Do You Want to Be Made Whole?," is designed to assist you in seven critical areas: (1) identifying your needs; (2) recognizing from whom you expect those needs to be met; (3) assessing the current status of getting those needs met; (4) recognizing how you feel when the needs are unmet; (5) identifying what you tend to do when these feelings accompany the unmet needs; (6) noting why you do what you do when the needs are unmet; (7) developing a strategy for addressing and meeting those needs.

Let's take a moment to address each point in the chart.

DO YOU WANT TO BE MADE WHOLE?

1	2	3	4	5	6	7
What Are My Needs?	From Whom?	Current Status	How I Feel When This Need Is Unmet	Manifested Behavior Pattern	Why?	Strategy
Acceptance	Family	Poor	Angry	Shuts down emotionally	Learned family behavior	Confrontation
Sense of accomplishment	Workplace	Good	Low self-esteem	Get behind in my work	Fear	Documented successes
Respect	Community	In progress	Isolated	Procrastination	Desire to be included	Grass-roots involvement

1. *What Are Your Needs?* Take time to answer this pivotal question. It's a question so many of us have avoided. Why? Because we have trained ourselves to not expect our needs to be met. The pain of asking and not receiving—the threat of rejection!—has been unbearable. As a result our pain is internalized and the freedom and the "license to ask" have been revoked in many folks' minds. You have a right, and a responsibility, to ask yourself: What are my needs? You cannot know yourself without taking and having an honest assessment of your

needs. You'll notice that in the chart I have identified as an example three needs of the average person: acceptance; a sense of accomplishment; and respect. Your needs may differ from these three; the important thing is to recognize them and write them down!

2. *From Whom Do You Expect Your Needs to Be Met?* Using the acceptance example in the chart, you may need acceptance from more than one community, person, or social unit. But, in this case, the person had identified that he or she primarily needs acceptance from his or her family. In column 2, write down all of the persons or social units from whom you expect to have your identified needs met.

3. *What Is the Current Status of Getting Your Needs Met?* This column gives you an opportunity to offer an honest assessment of the current status of how well your needs are being met. Allow me to offer four simple grading categories: good, poor, average, and in-progress.

4. *How Do You Feel When This Need Goes Unmet?* This column is designed to give you some insight into what is slowing you on your path to becoming whole. This will require some self-analysis, which, of course, is never easy. The devil loves to suppress emotions and feelings when disappointment clouds your head or heart. In the chart, I've shown a person who experiences a sense of anger when he is not accepted by his or her family, a sense of low self-esteem when he or she doesn't experience a sense of accomplishment in the workplace, and a sense of isolation when he or she doesn't feel respect from the community. But in spite of these perceived shortcomings, if you've isolated these feelings, you'll be well on your way to becoming whole, simply because you understand your needs. You'll no longer be in denial about your needs or from what or whom you expect to have those needs met. Most significantly, you'll know how you feel when your needs go unmet and you'll realize that these feelings stem from unmet needs and not ingrained deficiencies.

5. *What Is Your Behavior Pattern When Your Needs Aren't Met?* Knowing how you feel when your needs are unmet by certain persons or social

units is crucial because it's important to identify the relationship between emotions resulting from unmet needs and accompanying behavior patterns associated with the manifestation of these unmet
needs. For instance, when the person in our chart is not accepted and
feels angry, he or she habitually engages in self-destructive behavior.
Others may go on shopping sprees. Others may go on drinking, gam-
bling, smoking, or adultery binges. Others may contemplate suicide.
Others may become verbally or physically violent. Others may make
foolish business decisions regarding their economic future. Others
speak beyond their boundaries, then need to seek forgiveness from
those they've insulted or slandered. The important thing is to know
how you act out your unmet needs! When you feel isolated, angry, or
unloved, what do you do? What is your behavior pattern? What patterns have you attached to certain negative emotional experiences?
Identify them and write them down!

6.   *Why Do You Do What You Do?* On the path to wholeness, it's critical
     that you understand yourself. In order to understand yourself, you
     need some authentic working knowledge of why you do what you
     do. In other words, of all of the incredibly vast spectrum of emotions
     available to your psyche, why do you choose or gravitate toward cer-
     tain particular feelings or manifestations? Self-knowledge is power!
     As we've discussed, you do not want the devil to know more about
     yourself than you do.

7.   *What Is Your Strategy for Addressing the Unmet Need Expressed in Column
     #1?* Ask yourself these questions: How should I approach the person
     or persons from whom I expect my needs to be met (column 2)? How
     do my negative emotions manifest themselves? (column 5)? What am
     I going to do about this behavior pattern (column 7)? Once your strat-
     egy is formulated, determine who needs to be informed of your new
     boundaries, rules, focus, and direction. This is going to involve some
     risk. For example, if the person in our chart has decided to approach
     those family members who have rejected him and tell them how their

rejection has hurt him and inquire about what he can do to be accepted, then he's going to risk rejection. But once you know what
needs have to occur in your life for you to find the acceptance for
which you're yearning, a major change will occur. The ball will be in
your court, and not in the court of extenuating circumstances. You can
either stay in the same place or move forward. It will be your choice.
In this way, you will be exercising leadership, control over your life.
You'll be one step closer to not allowing someone else to control you
long-distance by "jerking your chain" of anger via lack of acceptance.

Ultimately, you're responsibile for feeling accepted, having
healthy self-esteem, and feeling enfranchised, regardless of what
folks in your family, workplace, or community think, say, or do.
Accordingly, if you identify and express your feelings to the appropriate people and you get the response you'd expect from a statue
or a telephone pole, then be prepared to develop a strategy whereby
God can bless you, and you can bless yourself, independent of your
social environment.

Somebody reading this book is asking, "Why not develop this
initially and forgo communicating with the folks in Column 2, the
folks you expect to meet your needs? Who needs the hassle or the
risk of rejection?" That's a good question and a good point. Living
a life of isolation, however, is tantamount to living no life at all.

Becoming whole means becoming whole in your marriage,
family, community, and world. When you're whole, you'll live each
day as if it were your last. When you're whole, you'll treat your
spouse, family members, coworkers and neighbors as if each day
were their last. When you're whole, you live completely. So when
death comes, the devil will find no ax to grind in your head or your
heart. There will be no blood—no unfinished business or unresolved emotional issues—on your hands.

Becoming whole is a process. Each step offers deliverance,

growth, and integrity. There are no shortcuts or easy exits. The very essence of wholeness is "going all the way." Are you prepared for the journey? *Do you want to be made whole?*

PIECES IN SEARCH OF A WHOLE

Standing before our congregation, I can see the glories of Holistic Salvation, through hundreds of individuals who have said "Yes!" to the call, then walked defiantly toward the goal of becoming whole.

Of course, the Windsor Village you encountered at the beginning of this book has been transformed. The cobwebs are gone; the empty pews are overflowing; the land around the sanctuary, once for sale, is now part of but one parcel owned by our Church. The success that some thought was reserved for the spiritually deficient has been harnessed. We have identified our needs, developed a strategy for getting those needs met, reclaimed our God-given destiny, and we are making ourselves whole.

Every Sunday, I stare out at the congregation of sanctified souls and see people who are secure in the knowledge that God didn't create anything—or anybody—halfway.

I see young men like Ali, twenty-four, named for his father's hero, Muhammad Ali. For years, he was a victim of what we refer to at Windsor Village as living in a Pig Pen. This is a place where so many of us reside, some for a short time, others for a lifetime. The Pig Pen is where life is shattered into so many pieces that a person is literally slopping around in the muck and the mayhem, his or her needs buried deep beneath the rubble. "I was just out there, taking whatever came my way," says Ali. Whether it was jobs or dates or friends or money, he took whatever came in his life, never planning, never knowing of God's Divine plan for his life, just getting by. But then, one day, Ali defiantly climbed out of that Pig Pen and took an inventory, then control over his life, revitalizing every area of his existence. He realized he had been made whole.

I see bright career folks like Trevor, who was once torn by his love of what he saw as a successful "lifestyle." Yes, he had the Mercedes and the BMW and the models on his arm, with whom he'd fly off to New Orleans for midweek lunches. A piece of his life— "Following the Green God," he calls it—overshadowed every other aspect. He had been led to believe that he needed status and material things to be *somebody*. Not until he stepped outside of his preconceptions could he realize that his life was fractured and his genuine needs had long been going unmet. This crucial realization jump-started for him the process of becoming whole.

From that pulpit, I see women like Charlotte, who was "falling apart at the seams," as she puts it, each part of her life as shattered and jagged as shards of broken glass. Professionally, she was laid off. Relationally, she was a "challenged mother" to her teenage daughter and the long-suffering mate to a materially wealthy man with whom, she knew, she had absolutely nothing in common. Emotionally, she was battered. Spiritually, she was without a Church home and without a relationship with her Lord. She was so lost that one night she cried out, *"God, where are You?"*

It was a pivotal moment. After crawling out of the clouds of denial, she could see her needs clearly. Only then could she go about the process of realizing her wholeness. With the support of various ministries and workshops, she found her Calling as a writer, got a new job, met and married the love of her life, took her relationship with her daughter to a new level of love and trust . . . in short, she totally realigned the pieces of her life into a vessel that, she says, God constantly fills with blessing after blessing after blessing.

As I stand on that pulpit and stare out at that sea of faces, I see not only individuals made whole but a community that has also become one. I see a congregation of diverse individuals who, by bonding together under God's anointing, have created wonders none of us could have created alone. We eventually discovered that our wholeness as a congregation was a part of God's primary will. Knowing God's will is one thing; walking it out is entirely different! We had to "walk our talk" to receive our blessings. That walk has led us to increasingly higher summits. Once we identified our needs—and began developing strategies for getting those needs met—God began stepping up our blessings in direct proportion to our Faith. As our faithfulness grew, so did our opportunities to become more faithful. Unto whom much is given, much is expected. Once you get to one level, God is ready to move you up to the next.

We got tangible proof of this during a real estate transaction last year. Some folks might have called it a miracle. It is one more example of God's grace in action. I mentioned earlier that Evander Holyfield agreed to donate $1.2 million to begin construction of our prayer center. For three years, we searched for land upon which the prayer center could be built. We knew our need for the prayer center. We had developed a strategy to get that need met. But we couldn't find the land! We were searching and searching, and praying and praying. When you pray, God will direct your path. He might cut off one path, only to open up another. Finally, we found a piece of prime property at the corner of South Post Oak and West Orem.

I asked our real estate agent to identify the owner and inquire about the selling price.

"You own some property at the intersection of South Post Oak and West Orem," I eventually told the landowner. "We'd like to buy half of it."

"I'm sorry," he replied. "Number one, it's not for sale. Number two, if I were to sell it, I'd want to sell *all* of it, not half of it."

"But we do not have a need for two hundred thirty-four acres of land!" I said.

God knew better. God was leading us into a place that we didn't have the foresight to see on our own. After months of negotiation, we finally closed the deal. We now own *all, not half of,* 234 acres of land! Our needs grew in direct proportion to our Faith, and our Faith is constantly growing. On half of our land, we're going to develop Corinthian Pointe, a single-family residential subdivision with 440 single-family homes. Corinthian Pointe Commercial Park, a 8.5-acre commercial tract, will be home to several local and national stores. Across the street will be the prayer center donated by Evander Holyfield, catfish ponds, a comprehensive wellness center, a community park, a 15-plus-acre community garden, a continuum-care facility, and other enterprises conducive to creating social capital.

Trust combined with prayer is like throwing a rock in the middle of a pond. The rock lands at one point, but it has a rippling effect. We started out with prayer and now we've got a commercial development and a single-family residential subdivision and all sorts of other awesome blessings from God. Our congregation has become the embodiment of God's blessing of Good Success. We are, in short, realizing our wholeness as we identify and meet the needs of the community.

I am yet another seeker in that congregation, of course, one more traveler who said "Yes!" to the path to Good Success, one more human being who eventually recognized that every seemingly incongruent step of my life was part of God's primary will. I was, of course, the up-and-coming bond broker: one piece of me desiring that 280-Z 2+2 sports car and deliverance to the Promised Land of a six-figure income, the other piece inexorably pulled toward God's path. Only when I identified my needs—putting God first, making a contribution to the community—could I truly realize my wholeness.

One single, yet pivotal step—walking away from my so-called dream job and into the ministry—set me upon the path that would eventually bring me peace, healing, identity. As I said before, I didn't know where I was headed in the beginning. But I sure do now. I was headed toward a place where I would receive God's greatest glory: the place where I would realize I had been created whole, the place where I could add the greatest value to the community.

I hope that you, too, will soon make this incredible realization.

SIX STEPS TO SALVATION

"He who overcomes shall inherit all things."
—REVELATION 21:7

Every journey toward Holistic Salvation begins with a single, crucial step. Don't expect a yellow brick road or some sunlit passageway through the clouds. It is more than likely to come as a single, simple decision. The important thing is to take the step and begin the walk.

If you're unsure of your direction, study the six steps presented in this book. They will ideally help you find it. Remember, God plants seeds, but we have to first notice that He has planted them, and then we have to nurture them to make them grow. Now you know the six steps of Holistic Salvation, it's time to embark upon the journey toward wholeness.

Let's review those steps now:

1. *Find Your Calling*
2. *Stage a Comeback*
3. *Embark Upon a Faith Walk*
4. *Whup the Devil*
5. *Create Wealth God's Way*
6. *Learn—and Practice—the Fundamentals of God-Blessed Relationships*

The path to good success is calling you now. Say "Yes!" Do not deny, doubt, or delay.

You were put on this earth to accomplish a powerful purpose: to fulfill God's primary will for your life and to become a tremendous blessing to God, others, and yourself.

May God bless you in your journey and may you achieve the life and good success that God has already commissioned in your name:

May you become whole.

Acknowledgments

THIS BOOK IS A RESULT OF MANY FOLKS' PRAYERS, ENCOURAGE-
MENT, financial contributions, and personal sacrifice of time. John
S. Mbiti, the noted philosopher, once wrote, "I am because we are,
and because we are I am."

This book is because of a lot of "We's."

I love my Windsor Village Church family! Thank you for both
the prayer capital and economic capital you invested in a Vision
called The Power Center. You sacrificed when the building was
just an eyesore and The Power Center was an embryo of thought.
Thank you all very much.

Donald Bonham and Fiesta Mart, Inc.: You pulled the trigger
on this now internationally acclaimed community project by do-
nating the 104,000-square-foot buildings and the 25 acres of land
upon which The Power Center now sits. Your commitment to the
community deserves a hefty standing ovation. My utmost appreciation is also extended to Buster Friedman, Fiesta's commercial real
estate consultant, who helped me "plead my case."

A leader is only as effective as his or her board and executive director. Genora, J. Otis, Mrs. Collins, Al and Tina Z. . . . thank you,
thank you, thank you! Your indefatigable commitment and price-
less advice will always be a part of The Power Center's foundation.

Partnerships propelled us. Our partners in The Power Center
include the Windsor Village Church Family, Pappas Restaurants,
Houston Endowment, the M. D. Anderson Foundation, the
Hoglund Foundation, the Southwestern Bell Foundation, Anita

and Gerald Smith, Houston Community College, Chase Bank of Texas, the University of Texas Health Science Center–Memorial Hermann Healthcare System, Alpha Eyecare, The Power Center Pharmacy, the WIC Program, WAM, Inc., and the Imani School. Individuals from these entities believed in the Vision and are striving to deliver wholeness to both individuals and the community at large. Thanks! Thanks! Thanks!

Sister Norman, thank you for telling me there was a book inside of me when I did not see it or know it.

Doris Cooper, thank you for insisting and encouraging me during the "Shall I pursue this book stuff?" process. Your role was undeniably pivotal.

C.M., thank you for your steadfast support.

F.W.J.J., thank you for your "How's it going, partner?" encouragement.

Rick Wartzman, thanks to you and *The Wall Street Journal* for printing the front-page story about The Power Center. When you write, publishers read and respond.

I am most thankful to Dr. Henry Masters and the Hamilton Park Church Family and Dr. Earl Allen and the St. Mary's Church Family for helping me clarify my calling and offering employment.

I am also thankful to the Mount Vernon United Methodist Church for helping me to interpret my Faith Walk during my development years.

Bob Barnett, you're the best agent on either side of the Mississippi River. Thanks for representing me.

Diana Newman of Simon & Schuster, your patience, professionalism, and polite persistence have been invaluable! After reading the front-page story about The Power Center in *The Wall Street Journal,* you contacted me, excited over the idea of my writing a book, and wrote the book's original outline. Cherise, thank you for propelling this project across the finish line. The discernment, sensitivity, and commitment you invested in the book were most timely and highly valued. Thank you, Diana, Cherise, and everyone at Simon & Schuster, for honoring me as an author.

To the Church members who sacrificed their time, talent, and privacy to be interviewed by Mark Seal, thanks! The book would have lacked *umph!* without you.

Speaking of Mark, what a collaborator! God anointed you to work with me on this project. My hectic schedule, writer's blocks, and seemingly incessant "I'll get it to you tomorrow's" would have driven the average awesome collaborator crazy. Your humor, unbelievably ever-present pleasant disposition, and acumen were a real blessing to me. Thanks! I pray we can do it again!

Finally, thanks to you, the reader. I hope that this book blesses you. Thank you for purchasing and reading it. May you become whole.

About the Author

KIRBYJON H. CALDWELL, a native Houstonian, was educated in the Houston public schools and earned a bachelor of arts in economics from Carleton College in May 1975, a master's in business administration in finance from the University of Pennsylvania's Wharton School of Business in May 1977, a master's in theology from Southern Methodist University–Perkins School of Theology in December 1981, and an honorary doctor of laws from Huston-Tillotson College in October 1994.

In June 1981, Pastor Caldwell was appointed Associate Pastor at St. Mary's United Methodist Church in Houston, while completing his master's degree in theology. In June 1982, he was appointed Senior Pastor of the Windsor Village United Methodist Church. In September 1992, Pastor Caldwell was appointed Senior Pastor of St. John's United Methodist Church.

Pastor Caldwell and the community-outreach ministries of Windsor Village have been featured in several publications, including the *Wall Street Journal, U.S. News & World Report,* and *Fortune,* and are currently featured in the "Speak to My Heart" exhibit at the Smithsonian Institution in Washington, D.C. Additionally, *Newsweek* identified Pastor Caldwell as a member of the Century Club, *Newsweek*'s list of 100 people to watch as America prepares to pass through the gate to the next millennium.

Kirbyjon H. Caldwell is married to Suzette Turner Caldwell. They are the parents of Kirbyjon "Turner" Caldwell.

You can contact Pastor Caldwell and the Windsor Village United Methodist Church at

Windsor Village United Methodist Church
6000 Heatherbrook
Houston, TX 77085
(713) 723-8187
www.kingdombldrs.com